'Excoriatingly raw and honest. Dean [...] nation of the cost of his psychological wounds on his family, and especially his heroic wife, Mary. In diving into the science of PTSD and the philosophy of "moral injury", Yates brings fresh new insights for anyone who has been on this journey. I wish I'd read it sooner.' Hugh Riminton, National Affairs Editor for Network Ten and author of *Minefields: A Life in the News Game*

'I treat people with PTSD and I have anxiety. I found this astonishing account of trauma and its profound repercussions so immersive and real that I felt I was in the therapy space with Dean. His searing honesty in recounting the personal and family cost of living with a complex mental health issue made me incredibly emotional – as it will you.' Dr Mark Cross, psychiatrist, author of *Anxiety* and co-author of *Changing Minds*

'A gripping read that exposes the shocking holes in our health system when it comes to the treatment of PTSD. Dean's battle with his employers and insurance companies is a familiar story that needs our nation's attention. This book will resonate with all first responders, including war journalists. I praise Dean's raw honesty!' Senator Jacqui Lambie

'A story like no other. Dean's remarkable honesty and extraordinary personal journey is a gift to those who feel shackled by shame and defeated by trauma.' Peter Whish-Wilson, Greens Senator for Tasmania

'Put on your seatbelt before reading this. Dean Yates has produced the roughest, and most honest, journalistic memoir of war I've ever encountered.' Thomas E. Ricks, author of *Fiasco* and *Waging a Good War*

'*Line in the Sand* might have started as a personal odyssey, but along the way, Dean has produced a world class guidebook to the cutting edge of how we deal with traumatic wounds. This should be a textbook for everyone working in mental health, and an inspiring read for anyone who cares about taking light into the darkness.' Steve Biddulph AM, author of *Raising Boys, The New Manhood* and *Fully Human*

'A guiding light. Dean's book will allow others to search through and travel along this inspiring passageway with its difficult turns. It is not just a personal story but also brings a broader understanding of what treatment involves and the people he met along the way, especially veterans and first responders. It is a book that will engage and encourage readers from many different backgrounds.' Sandy McFarlane AO, Emeritus Professor of Psychiatry, University of Adelaide

'Dean Yates captures the after war of PTSD and moral injury in the most searing way . . . we desperately need to hear his story and to share it. Too moving for words.' Nancy Sherman, *New York Times* notable author

'No one knows more about the lies and deceit behind the events of Collateral Murder than Dean Yates and for the first time we understand fully the ongoing trauma for so many involved. Yates is ensuring with this book that one of the most deceitful acts of the Iraq war will not be forgotten as he dives headlong into the story of the murders of his colleagues in his bid for justice for all.' Lisa Millar, ABC journalist and presenter and author of *Daring to Fly*

'*Line in the Sand* is a story that courageously reveals the full spectrum of PTSD's impact – the collateral damage to intimate partners, family and friends enmeshed in the effect of trauma as it brutally plays out inside relationships. Dean Yates has levelled up his own vulnerability by fully reporting the disintegration of selfhood and its painful reclamation, giving survivors of trauma and the people that love them new insight and hope for recovery.' Dr Polly McGee, trauma therapist and author of *The Good Hustle*

'Dean Yates has written a brutally honest account of war and war reporting, battling within these pages, as he battles within himself, the myriad of demons war unleashes. His book is brilliant, heart-wrenching and lyrically written. It is destined to become a classic.' Chris Hedges, Pulitzer Prize-winning war correspondent for the *New York Times* and author of *War is a Force That Gives Us Meaning*

'This book might make for very uncomfortable reading, but that's why it's essential.' Geoff McDonald, global advocate, campaigner and consultant on mental health in the workplace

'Dean Yates bares his still healing heart and the depths of his humanity by providing a raw and utterly unguarded first-person account of the horrific losses and moral injuries he incurred as a correspondent covering wars and disasters, and provides a detailed equally raw description of the enormous psychological, emotional, physical, social, and spiritual aftermath of these experiences. Yates reveals an essential truth about recovery from trauma and moral injury, namely that it is a lifelong challenge, and it is never one thing. The most powerful feature of the book is Yates sharing his healing path, which was a combination of intensive journalistic self-reflection and knowledge-seeking, support-seeking, a family that stuck with him, caring connections, hearing about others painful paths, rituals in service of rebalancing the scales of his own essential goodness and the goodness of others, professional truth-telling and reconciliation, being valued and doing valuable things in the world to help others, and I suspect writing this heartfelt book.' Dr Brett Litz, co-author of *Adaptive Disclosure: A New Treatment for Military Trauma, Loss, and Moral Injury*

'Dean Yates' unsparing account of the impact of his psychological injuries on his family makes essential reading for anyone trying to understand the true cost of PTSD. This book is a clarion call for a new approach to preventing and treating trauma. A searing account of one journalist's battle to save his family – and himself – from the invisible injuries he brought home from war. Incendiary.' Matthew Green, author of *Aftershock: Fighting war, surviving trauma and finding peace*

'No work has ever pulled back the veil on the individual and family consequences of trauma and moral injury like this. Nothing is off limits in Dean's vivid description of how a career filled with trauma, epitomised by one incident, could completely impact every part of his life and his family. In his recovery, he found that there are so many others, including veterans, first responders and their families who have shared his dark journey. A journey characterised by overwhelming guilt and shame. Dean has so powerfully told many of their stories within his own.' John Bale, co-founder of Soldier On and Fortem and Afghanistan veteran

'In this raw, moving, and powerful book Dean Yates gives us an inside view of what it is like living with trauma and PTSD. This is a rare opportunity to feel the emotional journey of a mental illness and how it affects all aspects of a life. This book raises important questions about the impact work can have on an individual's mental health and the level of protection and support employees are given. It exposes the chasms into which individuals can fall unsupported and alone despite working in large organisations and surrounded by others.

Just for doing their jobs well.' Amy McKeown, award-winning workplace and mental health consultant

'Dean's frank account of the psychological toll of frontline journalism and the lack of institutional support for those affected by trauma is essential reading for anyone who wants to support journalists. What makes this memoir unique and compelling is the raw honesty with which Dean examines the impact his trauma had on his sexual desires, and how he justified these as part of a patriarchal understanding of relationships, which he came to question and revise in an effort to protect the woman he loves, save his marriage and keep his family together. Such honest unveiling is rare from men but of utmost importance when research shows that it is personal relationships and supportive familial bonds that are the most protective elements for mental health conditions.' Clothilde Redfern, Director of the Rory Peck Trust

'In *Line In the Sand*, Dean Yates has transformed his considerable journalistic skills from reporting on wars to witnessing our biggest struggle – the war within ourselves. As a leading journalist reporting from the warzones of the world, he inevitably experienced traumas and losses that resulted in PTSD and moral injury. Dean's book is an intense, gripping, courageous and naked account of his journey, struggles, and search for healing. It witnesses the culpability of our institutions in causing and prolonging trauma, the degree to which trauma impacts journalists and other violence-exposed professions, and the long and complex process needed for recovery and healing. *Line In the Sand* educates readers to this journey, its complexities, and the necessary inner work and social support needed for trauma healing.' Edward Tick, PhD and psychotherapist and author of *War and the Soul, Warrior's Return* and *Soul Medicine*

Dean Yates is a workplace mental health expert, public speaker, podcast host and journalist. He is an outspoken advocate on mental health, press freedom and government accountability.

Dean worked for 26 years at Reuters, the international news agency. He was bureau chief in Iraq, responsible for 100 people, and later head of mental health strategy from 2017 to 2020.

Dean lives in Evandale in Tasmania with his life partner Mary Binks and their three adult children, Patrick, Belle and Harry.

Line in the Sand

A life-changing journey through
a body and a mind after trauma

Dean Yates

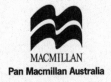

MACMILLAN
Pan Macmillan Australia

Pan Macmillan acknowledges the Traditional Custodians of country throughout Australia and their connections to lands, waters and communities. We pay our respect to Elders past and present and extend that respect to all Aboriginal and Torres Strait Islander peoples today. We honour more than sixty thousand years of storytelling, art and culture.

First published 2023 in Macmillan by Pan Macmillan Australia Pty Ltd
1 Market Street, Sydney, New South Wales, Australia, 2000

 A catalogue record for this book is available from the National Library of Australia

Typeset in 12.5/16.5 pt Adobe Garamond Pro by Post Pre-press Group

Printed by IVE

The author and the publisher have made every effort to contact copyright holders for material used in this book. Any person or organisation that may have been overlooked should contact the publisher.

Aboriginal and Torres Strait Islander people should be aware that this book may contain images or names of people now deceased.

Any health or medical content contained in this book is not intended as health or medical advice. The publishers and their respective employees, agents and authors are not liable for injuries or damage occasioned to any person as a result of reading or following any health or medical content contained in this book.

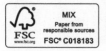 The paper in this book is FSC® certified. FSC® promotes environmentally responsible, socially beneficial and economically viable management of the world's forests.

For Namir Noor-Eldeen and Saeed Chmagh,
two men who told the truth about the Iraq War.

And for Mary, who fought a private war against PTSD and moral
injury, two illnesses that invaded and occupied the man she loves.

Contents

PART FOUR

'The sun made me squint. Twenty years. A lot like yesterday, a lot like never. In a way, maybe, I'd gone under with Kiowa, and now after two decades I'd mostly worked my way out. A hot afternoon, a bright August sun, and the war was over.'

Tim O'Brien, *The Things They Carried*
(Mariner Books, 1990)

PART ONE

PART ONE

1

Collateral Murder

Photographer Namir Noor-Eldeen makes his way through the al-Amin neighbourhood in eastern Baghdad looking for a story. In the mid-morning summer heat, raw sewerage leaks from broken pipes. Tangled electricity wires provide a few hours of power a day to Iraqi families behind their cracked mud-brick walls and metal gates.

It's 12 July 2007, the height of the Iraq War. Namir is a combat photographer for Reuters, the international news agency, and a veteran of the conflict at 22. He's checking out reports of a US air strike at dawn on a building in al-Amin's urban sprawl. With him is driver Saeed Chmagh, a 40-year-old father of four who knows the area well.

At 10.10 am, Namir gets in an abandoned car off an alleyway to photograph two women wearing traditional black garments and headscarfs walking towards a bullet hole in the windscreen. Who fired the shot is unknown. One woman, her arms outstretched, appears to be pleading with Namir. Her face is heavy with weariness. Below her palms, taking up the bottom half of the photo, is the bullet hole and cracked glass. The other woman's face is obscured. The woman with her arms extended looks like she is in mourning. In Iraq, every woman has lost someone to the war: a son, a daughter, a husband, a relative.

Namir and Saeed can't see or hear the two American AH-64 Apache helicopters prowling above the sand-coloured maze of al-Amin. A US infantry battalion searching for militias called them in after reports of sniper fire, gunmen on rooftops and rocket-propelled grenade (RPG) attacks on some of its soldiers. One of the Apaches has the call-sign Crazy Horse 1–8.

I'm in the Reuters office, a twenty-minute drive away. It's been more than four years since President George W. Bush ousted Saddam Hussein and then, with wilful neglect, left the people of Iraq open to unimaginable horror. The previous weekend I wrote stories about suicide bombers and sectarian death squads who killed 250 people across Iraq. As bureau chief of the largest foreign news organisation in Baghdad, I fear for the safety of my staff more than anything. The Cradle of Civilisation is the most dangerous country on earth, ancient Baghdad the epicentre of this hellscape. Suicide bombers on foot, in cars and trucks, detonate themselves and their vehicles on the streets and in marketplaces every day. Some attacks rattle our office windows. Dozens of bodies are found each morning by roadsides, in ditches or in the Tigris River that winds through the city.

Reuters covers the war from a two-storey house the company has rented since Saddam's downfall. We employ nearly 100 Iraqi journalists and support staff across the country. Seven or eight foreigners and fifteen Iraqis sleep in three nearby houses, the windows padded with sandbags. The Iraqis have moved in over the years because their lives have been threatened or their neighbourhoods are too dangerous. Some have sent their families across the border to Syria or Jordan. Concrete blast walls 3.5 metres high surround each house. Iraqi guards with AK-47 assault rifles are posted at metal gates built into each wall and checkpoints at either end of the street. The *New York Times*, the BBC and the Associated Press news agency rent houses near us and are similarly protected. Our defacto media compound is located on the eastern side of the Tigris, which splits Baghdad roughly in half. We are in the so-called Red Zone, the name for the city outside the heavily fortified Green Zone, an enclave for Iraq's fractured leadership, the American embassy and the headquarters of the US military.

I can see most of the office from where I sit on the ground floor. I'm unaware of Namir's whereabouts, which is routine. I trust my senior TV and pictures staff. If they had to get my approval for every movement, we'd never report anything. A diesel-fuelled generator the size of a small truck rumbles from the yard outside, an incessant reminder that electricity is precious in Baghdad. It can hit 50 degrees Celsius in summer: crushing, life-sapping heat. A low hum of noise rises from the city, one of the largest in the Arab world, home to 6–7 million people. Outside my window, minarets pierce the skyline. Satellite dishes, banned under Saddam, dot the flat roofs of houses and buildings. Leaves from an occasional date palm add a dash of colour to an otherwise yellow dullness.

At 10.19 am Namir and Saeed join a dozen men along a street where a flat-bed trailer and other vehicles are parked in an open square filled with rubbish. The Apache helicopters spot the group using powerful optics technology. An onboard camera records every step the men on the ground take. A few are carrying AK-47s and what looks like an RPG launcher, all pointed down. The men walk casually. Namir and Saeed are not wearing flak jackets with PRESS markings or protective helmets because al-Qaeda and other militant groups deliberately kidnap and kill journalists.

Namir walks ahead with an unarmed man towards a walled compound on a street corner. The man gestures, like he wants to show Namir something.

Apaches resemble war machines from the *Terminator* movies. Just rotors and weapons. An M230 chain gun loaded with 30mm armour-piercing rounds swivels between the main landing gear. An Apache has a two-man crew, a pilot and gunner.

'Hotel 2–6, Crazy Horse 1–8. Have five to six individuals with AK-47s. Request permission to engage,' says the Crazy Horse 1–8 gunner in a matter-of-fact voice, using the call-sign of the infantry battalion below.

'Roger that. Uh. We have no personnel east of our position. So, uh, you are free to engage, over,' comes the reply.

Engage means attack, kill.

Houses block Crazy Horse 1–8's line of sight. It will have to do a loop. About twenty seconds later, Namir peers around the street corner with his long-lens camera raised. Crouched down, he takes four photographs of US Humvees from the battalion crossing the road, about 100 metres away.

'He's got an RPG,' the Crazy Horse 1–8 gunner says, agitated now.

Namir rejoins the men as they walk back in the direction they came. Saeed is a little further ahead, talking on his phone. Crazy Horse 1–8 needs another 40 seconds to get in position.

'Light 'em all up!' says the pilot.

The chain gun explodes into life at 10.21 am. While it can

shoot 300 rounds a minute, the gunner fires several short bursts. The rounds are the size of a small soft-drink bottle, the length of a man's hand, and fragment on impact. Most of the men fall to the ground in clouds of dust. Namir reacts more quickly than the others, fleeing to his left. The gunner tracks Namir as he runs, bent over, across a large pile of garbage. He drops into the waste, probably hit. He looks up in the direction of the fusillade. Maybe he sees the helicopter in those last seconds before his body shudders off the ground from more shells and disappears in dirt and rubbish.

Saeed also gets away initially and is moving fast along a walled compound, trying to use it for cover. Crazy Horse 1–8 spots Saeed and opens fire. He too is shrouded in dust.

The Apache shoots again at the main group of bodies.

'Oh, yeah, look at those dead bastards,' says the gunner.

'Nice,' replies the pilot.

All the men are dead, except Saeed, lying near a kerb. For three minutes he tries to get up and crawl, but his left leg is badly wounded. The crew want to finish him off.

'Come on, buddy,' says the pilot.

'All you gotta do is pick up a weapon,' adds the gunner.

A faded turquoise minivan stops next to Saeed at 10.26 am. Driver Saleh Matasher Tomal, 43, is unarmed. Inside are his son Sayad, ten, and daughter Doaha, five. Tomal is taking them to school.

The crew tells the ground unit the van is 'possibly' picking up bodies and weapons and requests permission to attack again. Tomal gets out and opens the side cargo door. Two other men arrive and grab Saeed. They appear to be unarmed bystanders.

'Come on, let us shoot!' says the gunner.

The two bystanders put Saeed in the van.

Permission to attack is granted.

Crazy Horse 1–8 fires several bursts, 120 rounds in total.

'Oh yeah, look at that. Right through the windshield! Haha!' says the gunner.

It's 10.29 am. Saeed and Tomal are dead, and probably the other men as well.

Troops from the infantry battalion arrive several minutes later.

At 10.35 am, one soldier says: 'I've got, uh, eleven Iraqi KIAs [killed in action]. One small child wounded. Over.

'We need, we need, uh, to evac [evacuate] this child. Ah, she's got a, uh, she's got a wound to the belly.'

'Well, it's their fault for bringing their kids into a battle,' says the Crazy Horse 1–8 gunner.

'That's right,' replies the pilot.

Both of Tomal's children are wounded but survive.

—

I'm sitting at the bureau 'slot' desk. It's a fixed position in all big Reuters reporting operations, someone monitoring the news, on alert. My job is to write the lead story of the day, work with our Iraqi reporters, and coordinate coverage with television and pictures staff. A phone with a direct line to editors in London sits on the desk.

Al-Qaeda suicide bombers tend to strike early, when markets are crowded, or young men are lined up at police and army recruiting centres. It's been quiet across Iraq this morning. I don't think I've written a single word, unlike most days since I arrived from Jerusalem six months earlier.

February 3: Truck bomb kills 135, wounds 305 at Baghdad market.
February 12: Bombs ravage Baghdad markets, killing 88.
March 29: Suicide bombers kill 130 in Iraq.

March 31: Tal Afar bomb killed 152, deadliest of war.
April 18: Suspected al-Qaeda bombs kill nearly 200 near Baghdad.
June 19: Bomb kills 78 in Baghdad, US in big offensive.

Staff are working on feature articles. Catching up on admin. Chatting among themselves. I've been trying to kill flies around my desk with a plastic swatter. They drive everyone mad.

Suddenly, loud wailing breaks out at the back of the office, near a small room where the drivers relax and drink coffee. I stand up, heart pounding, senses primed. Something terrible has happened; the pitch of the anguish is not of this earth. A young Iraqi cameraman bursts through the door. I'll never forget the horror and pain on his face, his hands clutching his head. He speaks rapidly in Arabic. A senior Iraqi journalist sitting next to me has also gotten up.

'Namir and Saeed have been killed,' he translates. 'Possible US helicopter attack.'

I walk towards them, trying to ignore the tightness in my chest. Staff are pouring into the newsroom, shouting in Arabic. I can't show emotion, I need to show leadership.

'Let's get all the information we can,' I say.

Colleagues try Namir's phone but it keeps ringing out. Saeed's appears to be switched off or isn't working. Several photographers and cameramen get in cars and rush to al-Amin. I take a few deep breaths and call Michael Lawrence, the global news editor in London, somehow keeping my voice under control: 'I've got terrible news. It looks like two Iraqi staff have been killed.'

A photographer finds Namir's body in a hospital morgue with no electricity. He and Namir were close friends, lived in the same house in the compound. At night they lay on their beds and talked about photography and what they would do after the war.

The photographer packs Namir's body with ice. I can't remember who found Saeed.

People in al-Amin tell my staff a US helicopter attacked a group of men that included Namir and Saeed. US soldiers took Namir's cameras, they said, which means we can't review what he'd been photographing. I email the US military spokesman for Iraq, a one-star general in the Green Zone. I want everything in writing, and I figure he can get me answers fast. I've met him a few times and like him. He's smart and friendly. He replies to my email quickly, saying he will check.

The bureau is in full-scale crisis now. Many staff are wailing. Because my partner Mary Binks follows events in Iraq from our home in Australia, I text her: 'Think two of my staff have just been killed.' It's evening at the house we rent in rural bushland north of Sydney. Mary will always remember what she was doing because it was so discordant with the tragedy unfolding in Baghdad: she and our three young children – Patrick, Belle and Harry – were dancing to a Justin Timberlake song in the kitchen. Mary, a former journalist, has also lost colleagues to war.

I study the footage and photographs my staff bring back from the scene. They show bewildered residents standing next to a dusty turquoise minivan, its front torn off. There is a pool of blood near a kerb but no bodies. The road, pavement and walls are pockmarked by heavy calibre ammunition.

Residents say the van was near Namir and Saeed at the time and that other people were killed inside the vehicle. Two Irish security contractors who work for Reuters, both former members of the Royal Ulster Constabulary, watch the footage and say the van was probably hit by a missile. Iraqi police call the attack 'random American bombardment' and put the death toll at twelve. Nothing makes sense.

I get an email from a colleague at another foreign media organisation expressing sadness about Namir and Saeed but also wanting to confirm their deaths. Of course, this is news. More emails arrive asking the same question. All my foreign colleagues wait until I write a five-paragraph story before reporting the event. This makes it real, not a nightmare. Doing something I've done thousands of times for Reuters across Asia and the Middle East for fifteen years.

BAGHDAD, July 12, (Reuters) – An Iraqi photographer and driver working for Reuters in Iraq were killed in Baghdad on Thursday in what police said was American military action and which witnesses described as a helicopter attack.

The bureau arranges for Namir's body to be driven the next day to the northern city of Mosul, his birthplace. A few colleagues will travel with his coffin. Saeed's family will take his body to the holy Shi'ite city of Najaf, south of Baghdad. I get cash from the safe to give to both families for funeral and other expenses.

Do I pause at this moment to consider the risks we take as journalists? What price – in compensation – will Reuters put on the lives of Namir and Saeed? I can't recall.

The sheer amount of work keeps me focused: debriefing Iraqi reporters trying to find out what happened, supporting my staff and updating my editors in London.

More precisely, the work, the responsibility I carry, stops me falling apart.

By early evening the US military has still said nothing. I press the spokesman for comment and the return of Namir's cameras. The military is investigating, he says. I've updated the initial story twice. It's been twelve hours since Namir and Saeed were killed.

*

Just after midnight, the US military issues a statement, saying US forces returned fire and called in helicopter support after being attacked with small arms and RPGs.

'Nine insurgents were killed in the ensuing firefight. One insurgent was wounded and two civilians were killed during the firefight. The two civilians were reported as employees for the Reuters news service,' the statement says.

'There is no question that Coalition Forces were clearly engaged in combat operations against a hostile force,' says a spokesperson for US forces in Baghdad, a lieutenant-colonel.

The assertion that Namir and Saeed were killed in a firefight is a lie, but I don't know that yet. It will be the first of many lies the US military and government tells over the coming years about this terrible day, from a lieutenant-colonel in public affairs in Baghdad, to a US secretary of defense in Washington.

I update the story from my bedroom, reporting what the military has said. It's now 2 am. Condolence messages from around the world are flooding my inbox. The attack is one of the world's top stories.

Exhausted, I somehow manage to get a bit of sleep.

The next morning my distraught Iraqi staff help family members strap wooden coffins containing the bodies of Namir and Saeed to the top of two cars for a small funeral procession in Baghdad. As a foreigner, it's too dangerous for me to attend, even for a few minutes. Militants might spot me. It's risky also for the staff and families as suicide bombers often target funerals.

One photo shows the young Iraqi cameraman next to the car carrying Namir's coffin, wailing uncontrollably, gripping his head. Another shows Saeed's mother, dressed in black garments, collapsed on the ground next to the vehicle carrying her son's coffin.

In yet another, Saeed's eldest son, Salwan, fifteen, his face stricken with grief, clings to the car's roof racks.

A picture of Saeed is taped to the front of the coffin. The lid doesn't fit properly, not even close. Baghdad is a warzone, I know, coffin makers overworked, but it still seems a gross indignity.

I email the military spokesman again, asking for the immediate return of Namir's cameras and their disks. I request access to cameras from the US helicopters, as well as voice communications between the pilots and ground units.

The following day, an Iraqi translator called Lu'oy al-Joubouri doesn't show for work or call, which is unusual. Lu'oy has been with us since March and is always punctual. I ask reporter Aseel Kami to track him down. Aseel was a dressmaker before the US invasion. She joined Reuters as a translator in 2004, then became a reporter. Aseel is a stylish feminine presence in a largely male office. She softens the madness of Baghdad.

Aseel finally reaches Lu'oy's father. I watch her face turn ashen, then she hangs up and walks over to me. Lu'oy is dead, Aseel says. He and his two brothers were driving home on Wednesday – the day before Namir and Saeed were killed – when militants forced their car to stop near their parents' home and shot them. Maybe they demanded to see ID. The family name, al-Joubouri, is instantly recognisable as Sunni. The gunmen were presumably Shi'ite. Lu'oy, 30, had two young children.

Lu'oy's parents didn't know he worked for Reuters. Some staff don't want to worry their families. I write a short story without mentioning Lu'oy's name, respecting their wishes.

That evening, Mariam Karouny, a young Lebanese journalist who is my deputy, comes to my office and closes the door. I prefer to work in the open newsroom, but sometimes I need privacy. I've made little attempt to personalise my office apart from putting photographs of Mary and the children on the wall next to my desk.

Mariam, 27, has a deep understanding of the Iraq story. She can get government ministers on the phone when others can't. I think she intimidates them with the force of her personality. She was close to Namir, treated him like a younger brother. Namir's death has crushed her.

Mariam and I have built a strong working relationship over the past six months. Running a large operation in a warzone requires trust and honesty. Mariam tells me the Iraqi staff think I'm being too soft on the US military in our reporting about Namir and Saeed. They are angry, she says quietly. They want me to write that Namir and Saeed were killed in cold blood.

Caught off-guard, I try to process what Mariam has said. *Soft.* My staff are calling me a coward. I know they are grieving and want justice, but we must be balanced in our reporting: this goes to the heart of being a Reuters journalist, I tell Mariam. And I can only write what we know, which is little.

Despite the assurance I give her, something inside my body, my heart maybe, breaks. These Iraqi journalists, who I admire so much, who risk their lives every day, who've suffered immeasurable loss during more than four years of war, think I'm gutless, not on their side. The tough exterior I've worn all my life, the rock I've been for others, crumbles. I weep.

I can't do this. I can't do this.

Expecting me to be hurt but stunned by my emotion, Mariam comes over and hugs me tightly.

I've breathed in the ashes of a bombed nightclub in Bali; seen thousands of dead bodies after the most devastating tsunami in history; pushed myself to the limit covering earthquakes that no one will remember. But I'm not up to this. I don't want this responsibility. I want to call Michael Lawrence, resign, I tell Mariam.

'The stress is too much,' I say, my body trembling. 'Someone stronger needs to take over.'

'We need you. The bureau needs you,' Mariam replies. This young woman on her first foreign posting urges me to stay on, senses I'll never forgive myself if I quit. She probably saves my career. Bureau chiefs don't abandon their posts.

———

Ten days later I'm sitting opposite two American generals and a small TV monitor in a nondescript room inside Saddam's former Republican Palace in the Green Zone. The massive rectangular building was spared the invasion bombardment and is now headquarters to the US military, political and diplomatic presence in Iraq.

The military returned Namir's cameras a few days after he was killed. They haven't been tampered with, no photos deleted. The cameras show the women dressed in black, then, roughly ten minutes later, Humvees at a crossroad, quickly followed by the top of the head of someone who appeared to be falling as dust sprayed off a wall. No images of fighting or people running for cover. No gunmen. The next pictures, taken more than three hours later, are of an American soldier sitting in what looked like a tent or barrack. It is slightly out of focus.

Witnesses and residents I'd interviewed in the Reuters office said there hadn't been any clashes in that part of al-Amin to explain the helicopter strike, nor had they seen gunmen. It was obvious Namir and Saeed weren't killed in a firefight.

I forwarded the military spokesman a letter from the Reuters editor-in-chief on 16 July, demanding a full and objective investigation given the evidence the bureau had gathered casting doubt on the military's version of events. I wrote a story based on the letter. In the days that followed, as I interviewed more residents and reflected on Namir's final photographs, the words that kept forming on my lips were 'cold-blooded murder'. I've come to the Republican Palace, sitting in this small room, convinced my Iraqi staff are right. I'm also furious that just days ago the military sent heavily armed US and Iraqi troops unannounced to Namir's family home in Mosul while they were marking the 40-day Muslim mourning period. They wanted to see his death certificate, ripped down black mourning banners outside the home, asked neighbours if his family had ties to terrorists. What were they looking for? Justification for having killed Namir?

The spokesman ignored my angry email. Instead, he invited me to hear the results of the military's investigation into Namir and Saeed's deaths.

The briefing is off-the-record, which means I won't be able to report anything for Reuters. Michael Lawrence is next to me. A fellow Australian, he's flown in from London. We sit on one side of a table, two generals in desert camouflage uniforms on the other. No medals, just last names sewn above their right breast pockets and single pentagonal stars on their shoulders. The spokesman is an avuncular figure with greying hair and a moustache. The other general is tall, ten years older than me, a familiar face to anyone who has followed the fiasco of America's occupation of Iraq. He oversaw the investigation and does most of the talking.

He begins by saying that hundreds of soldiers from the

2nd Battalion, 16th Infantry Regiment had been operating in al-Amin since dawn on 12 July to clear out Shi'ite militias who had been setting off roadside bombs. After coming under attack from small-arms fire and RPGs, the 2–16 requested air support. Two Apaches arrived and spotted eight to ten men. The group formed, dispersed, then formed again, he said. They appeared to be 'conferring'. Some of the men could 'clearly' be seen carrying rifles and RPGs. Two other men also had something slung over their shoulders. From 9.45 am to 10 am, units of the 2–16 had come under fire elsewhere in al-Amin, he said. While no shooting came from the group that included Namir and Saeed, the 2–16 gave the Apaches clearance to attack.

What do you mean, Michael and I ask, no one fired on US forces? The presence of armed men was an expression of 'hostile intent' and thus the group could be 'engaged', the investigating general says. The military has rules of engagement (ROEs) for Iraq, parameters for the use of force based on the Law of Armed Conflict, a collection of international treaties such as the 1949 Geneva Conventions.

My head spins. *How can this be hostile intent? No one fired on US forces.* I don't know it yet, but the ROEs define hostile intent as the threat of imminent use of force, where imminent doesn't necessarily mean immediate or instantaneous. A commander just needs to *believe* an attack will occur.

An initial burst of fire from one Apache killed seven 'military-aged' men, the investigating general says. We are shown photographs of an AK-47, two RPGs and two cameras that he says were found within a 10-metre radius. The general shows us a written report with timestamps and conversations between the Apache crew. Michael and I again ask: Where is the hostile intent if no one fired on US forces? Carrying weapons is hostile intent, the general replies. Every house has an AK-47, I say. Yes, but not RPGs and even if they have AK-47s, it's against the law to have them on the street, the general says.

The investigating general then says he will show us footage from one of the Apaches.

I have little time to think before a TV a bit bigger than a shoebox flickers to life. It's a grainy black and white scene. I see the rooftops of al-Amin, a mosque, walled compounds clustered tightly together. The gunner alerts the pilot to the group of men. The Apache's camera zooms in and with deepening dread I recognise Saeed because he is a bit overweight and then Namir by the slightly bow-legged way he walks. They each have a camera over their shoulders. I see the flat-bed trailer and other vehicles. One of the other men has a long, cylindrical object pointed downward, which the investigating general says is an RPG. Two other men appear to have rifles, carried loosely by their side.

No US or Iraqi forces are visible. No firefight.

My heart races.

Crazy Horse 1–8 starts to circle.

Namir walks ahead, looks around a corner, crouches and points his long-lensed camera down a street.

'He's got an RPG,' the gunner says rapidly.

'Just fuckin', once you get on 'em, just open 'em up,' replies the pilot.

Seconds later Crazy Horse 1–8 is in position.

Cannon shells crash into the men.

The tape is stopped. I lean forward, head in my hands. I can't remember if Michael says anything, but I'm speechless. I can barely breathe.

Oh my God. Namir looked so suspicious.

The investigating general keeps talking.

Even if the crew determined Namir was pointing a camera at the Humvees, the helicopters would probably still have opened fire because insurgents filmed their attacks on US forces, he says. Such recordings were uploaded to the internet for propaganda purposes. The crouching, the peering around the corner, was also an expression of 'hostile intent'.

Further footage shows a minivan stopping to help the wounded, adds the investigating general. The driver was believed to be aiding insurgents, so the helicopter attacked again. Michael asks to see this footage. The generals refuse. Michael asks for copies of the video and photographs. Again, the answer is no. Michael even picks up the file the general has and asks if he can take it. Yet again, no. Reuters must make a request for the materials under the US *Freedom of Information Act* (FOIA) via the Pentagon.

The generals don't apologise for the 'firefight' lie or seek to explain. I'm too shocked to remonstrate. With no warning, we've just watched Namir and Saeed walk into their deaths. Less than three minutes of footage. Michael and I don't know what's on the rest of the tape, apart from the limited account we've been given of the minivan attack.

The meeting is over. We thank the generals and leave. I walk out of the Republican Palace into bright summer sunshine with one image seared into my brain: Namir peering around that corner.

Two days later I send an email marked confidential to the bureau chiefs of other foreign news agencies who, like Reuters, employ mostly Iraqi staff. I give them a lot of detail so they can better protect their teams. I suggest they share the information during a general chat about security. Please don't mention Namir and Saeed, I add.

The Apache crew was very suspicious of the group of men, I write. They saw gunmen and two men with 'objects' slung over their shoulders; Namir and Saeed both carried a camera. The Apache was told there were no US soldiers or Iraqi security forces near the group. What happened next was Namir could be seen walking to a small intersection, I write. My 600-word email omits the fact that Crazy Horse 1–8 got permission to open fire and was manoeuvring into position to shoot before Namir looked around the corner.

Just two days and I'm blaming Namir for the attack.

—

In late 2009, at a US military base near Baghdad, an army intelligence analyst called Chelsea Manning hears colleagues discussing a classified video. It's footage from the gun-camera of Crazy Horse 1–8 showing Namir and Saeed being killed. Manning has watched what she describes as 'countless war-porn type videos depicting combat' and isn't too interested until she sees Crazy Horse 1–8 open fire on the minivan. As her colleagues, officers among them, debate whether that attack violated the rules of engagement for Iraq, Manning wants to know more. She finds news stories on Namir and Saeed and the US government's refusal to give Reuters a copy of the tape. The strike on the minivan especially troubles her, as does the way the Crazy Horse 1–8 crew dehumanise the men on the ground as they speak.

Manning copies the tape and the ROEs, planning to give them to Reuters in London after her deployment ends, so the organisation has more context for what happened. In early 2010, she decides to send the material to an obscure anti-secrecy group called WikiLeaks instead so Reuters might get the information sooner.

Manning, 22, hasn't suddenly turned whistleblower. Dismayed at what she saw as the American public's lack of awareness of what was happening in Iraq, Manning has recently orchestrated the biggest leak of official secrets in US history: sending 700,000 classified documents to WikiLeaks about the wars in Iraq and Afghanistan, as well as US State Department cables and detainee assessment briefs from the Guantanamo prison camp. WikiLeaks hasn't done anything with those documents yet, but after analysing the footage of Namir and Saeed's deaths and researching the event it captured, the Australian founder of WikiLeaks, Julian Assange, knows he has a damning snapshot of how America wages war in Iraq.

Assange cuts a striking figure at the National Press Club in Washington on 5 April 2010. It's been nearly three years since Namir and Saeed were killed. Late 30s, slim, blond hair, Assange is little known outside computer hacker circles but will become one of the most recognisable men in the world after unveiling the video he famously calls 'Collateral Murder'. The footage horrifies people around the globe. International legal experts call the attack on the minivan that killed Saeed a war crime, a violation of the Geneva Conventions. Critics liken the pilot banter to teenagers playing video games. WikiLeaks puts a 17-minute edited version and the full 38-minute tape on the internet. The most controversial footage in the history of war is a mouse-click away.

While Assange is addressing the world's media in Washington, my family and I are asleep in a lodge in the Cradle Mountain National Park in Tasmania. The area is an alpine wonderland of ancient King Billy pines, icy streams and cabins warmed by wood-fired stoves. No mobile phone or data service, not even TV. Events have been set in motion that will shape the rest of my life.

On 7 April, we drive to Devonport on Tasmania's northwest coast to see Mary's parents. I don't turn on my phone. A couple of hours later I open a local newspaper. The Collateral Murder story is spread across the inside pages.

My jaw drops. This can't be. *Baghdad, 12 July 2007.* Then I see an image of Saeed taken from TV footage, wounded, trying to get up. I read the pilot chatter. My brain freezes.

They fucked us. The generals fucked us.

Fury is soon replaced by desolation. I failed Namir and Saeed. For reasons that will take years to understand, I say nothing publicly. That will compound my sense of failure and turn into deep, withering shame.

2

Rock bottom

Gravity presses the side of my head into the pillow. Saliva seeps from the corner of my mouth. I'm a husk of a man in a darkened room on a cold winter's evening in the village of Evandale in Tasmania.

A streetlight casts a faint glow through a gap in the heavy curtains. At the other end of a long hallway is the kitchen and living room, a chaotic mix of three teenagers, four cats and a dog. Our home sits among Georgian houses and colonial-era churches on a hill overlooking a flat expanse of green fields where a farmer grazes his sheep and cattle. From the living room we can see the South Esk River snaking through the paddocks. In the distance stand the Great Western Tiers, an unbroken line of mountain bluffs, occasionally snow-capped in winter.

It's 27 July 2016. Five months since a psychiatrist in Hobart diagnosed me with post-traumatic stress disorder; five months on sick leave; five months of plunging into an abyss. It's hard to stop falling when you don't understand why you fell in the first place.

*

Mary and I moved our family to Evandale three and a half years ago from Singapore. I was hollowed out after two decades of working overseas for Reuters. The bosses had agreed I could edit stories from wherever I made my home. I bought a book on fly-fishing in Tasmania, the beautiful island where Mary was born. I daydreamed of wearing green waders and casting for trout in rivers and streams. Only the sound of water and a fish breaking the surface. It wasn't long before Mary and the kids would freeze if anyone dropped something or slammed a door. They tried to second-guess my moods. Tiny things irritated me while depression sucked me dry. I'm not sure how they co-exist, but juxtaposed with an emptiness that sometimes flattened me was a volcanic anger that turned the house into a minefield for the people I love most in the world.

Dozens of sights and sounds began intruding into my head years ago. Intermittent at first, frequent now: the severed hand I almost trod on in the wreckage of the bombed Sari Club in Kuta Beach; the 158 bloated bodies I counted in the Baiturrahman Grand Mosque in Indonesia's Banda Aceh after the 2004 Boxing Day tsunami; the two South Korean contractors slumped dead in their car, ambushed on a lawless stretch of road in Iraq. The wailing at the back of the Reuters house in Baghdad. I never thought a man could sound so grief-stricken.

My nightmares started as soon as I went on sick leave.

Gunmen chase me through the streets of Baghdad. It's the height of the Iraq War; suicide bombers killing dozens every day; tens of thousands of American soldiers fighting insurgents for control of a mutilated city; Apache gunships unleashing hell from the sky. My toenails scratch the sheets and rustic wooden frame of our king-size Javanese bed, sometimes waking Mary. My feet move. I literally run. I have no physical bruises the next morning, but my insides are battered. It feels like someone has tossed me about the room. Even when I'm not being pursued in my sleep, the scenes are always violent. Beheadings. Bombings. US artillery strikes. I'm in Iraq or elsewhere in the Middle East. People I know sometimes appear, usually journalists. I also show up in Indonesia or Australia. Then there is lots of water, flooding. I must flee or drown.

My psychiatrist hasn't noticed how fast I've deteriorated. He can't see through the mask I wear at our monthly sessions. The well-dressed, articulate 47-year-old journalist sitting opposite him. Maybe I don't fit the profile of others who've come back from war; maybe I'm better at hiding how broken I am. He has me on a moderate dose of antidepressants, nothing else. I self-medicate with codeine, Xanax and Captain Morgan rum. Rest, my psychiatrist has said. Problem is – on sick leave and therefore free of editing copy, writing emails and taking part in daily news-planning calls – my mind has declared war on itself.

The psychiatrist hasn't recommended I see a therapist to process my trauma. During a recent session, Mary sat in a chair next to me in quiet frustration and anger while I played things down. Mary had wanted to talk to him alone after she feared I'd hit her during an outburst. She'd been determined the psychiatrist understand the truth of my condition. Instead, he stood at his door until I walked in. Another male doctor in his office observing 'for experience' said nothing.

No one from Reuters has called me. The bosses in the regional office in Singapore and headquarters in New York haven't even asked if I have the right treatment plan in place. Since I don't have one, it's sort of moot, but their indifference has gutted me. It's like I don't exist. The bosses haven't connected me with

25

an internal peer network of journalists who support distressed colleagues or suggest I talk with the company's external trauma service in London. These supports should be routine, especially given my experience: three staff killed on my watch. I've sent the bosses a couple of emails with updates on my mental state, but I don't call because my self-esteem has shattered into a thousand pieces. In any case, Reuters must reckon I'm damaged goods because in a few months, after my first admission to a psychiatric unit in Melbourne, the company will try to force me out.

—

As I lie in bed, Mary is in the kitchen preparing a meal after getting home from TAFE, where she is doing a Diploma in Community Services.

She will have lit the wood-fired heater in the living room. There is a story behind every piece of furniture in our bedroom, every print and painting on the wall.

I love and respect my intelligent and passionate partner. A fearless journalist for twenty years in Australia and Asia, Mary had been my inspiration. She showed me it was possible to cover dangerous stories and come back alive. If there was an envelope in sight, Mary pushed it. I wanted to emulate her. Mary gave me the courage to go to Baghdad in the first place.

I met Mary in the Reuters newsroom in mid-1995 in Hong Kong, where she was working as a reporter and a TV producer, and as a freelance journalist for *TIME* magazine. She was 32. I was 27. I'd just moved from Jakarta and was the most junior member of the Reuters Asia editing desk.

I was captivated the moment I saw Mary. I'd steal glances

at her; tailored jackets and knee-high boots, her long wavy blonde hair parted or tied back. A journalist for nearly fifteen years by then, Mary mixed worldly confidence with quirkiness and a playful smile. A big story was brewing with Hong Kong's return to China a couple of years away. Mary was all over it. She belonged. I was out of my depth.

Mary had poise, intelligence and strong convictions. Indonesia's occupation of East Timor was genocide, she told me. President Suharto a dictator. I tried to argue that Suharto's rule, while authoritarian and corrupt, had brought progress to Indonesia. Mary didn't buy it.

In Jakarta, I was close friends with young Indonesian journalists who worked at three publications banned by Suharto in 1994. I went to meetings of an illegal organisation they set up in a squalid apartment block behind the capital's glittering hotels and malls. My boss at the time said I was too close to the story. Maybe. But my passion was a candle flame compared to the inferno inside Mary.

She won a Walkley Award for her coverage of Tasmania's Forest Wars for a local newspaper, aged 24. Mary was never cowed by intimidation from the state's political and business interests who hated her stories – all men, of course.

One evening in 1999, as we sat on a beach in Bali, Mary nagging the Reuters TV editors to let her go to East Timor as pro-Jakarta militias rampaged following an independence vote, she said it was worth dying for such an important story.

I'd never met a woman like her: tough and independent but also soft and feminine. Mary's desire and tenderness awoke senses in me I didn't know existed. I think I knew Mary was The One the first night we spent together in Hong Kong. She took some convincing I was the one for her, though.

Mary also knew mental illness, having first experienced debilitating depression at seventeen following the sudden death of a childhood friend. That tragedy triggered memories of childhood trauma for Mary. At high school for a month or so after her friend died, during every break, she shut herself in a tiny windowless study room in the library because she couldn't face people. She tried to take her own life. Some days as a reporter in Hobart, Mary sat at her desk and stared at the phone, unable to lift the receiver. She had a broken marriage in her twenties and was diagnosed with depression at 30.

Mary's illness bewildered me when she was so depressed she couldn't speak. But these episodes were few because she understands her depression. She takes her medication and has the self-awareness to let me know if she is feeling low. I can also usually sense when she is unwell.

But *my* mental health? No, Mary was wrong during those years when she urged me to get help. I'm fine, I kept telling her.

After what I coped with at Reuters, mental illness was unfathomable, not part of my identity. Besides, it had been ages since I was in a warzone. The other thing that stopped me from listening to Mary was my masculinity, my manhood.

After my diagnosis, I felt no emotion, nothing. I had a name for my condition, but no relief. Mary persuaded me to a do an eight-week mindfulness course, hoping it might ease my anxiety and agitation. I liked the practice, but the best therapy, or so I thought, came from hiking in the Tarkine rainforest in Tasmania's northwest.

My days at home were aimless. Patrick, Belle and Harry had always seen me put in long hours, often travelling. They knew I worked on big stories. Suddenly, they saw their dad in the living room, staring into space, or watching TV, day after day. I didn't notice their growing anxieties, their struggles at school, sense their wariness, their confusion about the changes in me. Mary loves me despite what I've become. Despite the things I did that could have destroyed the life we built together. I love Mary in my head but feel little in my heart. I'm numb.

Trauma is like a cluster bomb. Everyone around you gets hurt.

——

Patrick, fifteen, was sick yesterday but I cancelled his doctor's appointment. Like now, I couldn't get out of bed. Mary was at TAFE. We adopted Patrick from an orphanage in Jakarta when he was fifteen months old and nicknamed him Paddy. Reuters had asked me to return to Indonesia the previous year. He'd often put his tiny feet into my brown R.M. Williams boots when I'd get home from work and try to run. He'd trip over, giggling. Later, aged seven, Patrick saw me doing a live TV interview from the roof of the Baghdad office and burst into tears. Black smoke billowed in the background from a car bombing, several kilometres away. Patrick thought I was in danger. Unlike many teenage boys who resist a parental embrace, Patrick loves being hugged. It's not that I don't put my arms around him anymore. He just senses I'm not there. He's been depressed and absent from school.

Harry, thirteen, feels the torment I seem able to express only in my journal. He has severe anxiety, missed a lot of school this year. Harry told me he knows I risked my life in Iraq. I think it's his way of acknowledging the weight I carry. If only he didn't have to carry it too. Harry and I were sitting at the kitchen table last week when our dog barked near me. I slammed my hand on the table and flew at the dog. Right arm raised, fist clenched, I stopped myself just in time. I thought my heart would blast out of my chest. I went to bed. I don't remember saying anything to Harry.

When Mary gave birth to Harry in Singapore six weeks after the Bali bombings, I wanted to get away from the hospital and back to Jakarta. I missed the newsroom noise, the pull of a big story. I couldn't sit with my baby and my partner. I didn't shed a tear of joy. Mary noticed but didn't say anything. I can still see Harry's eyes on me when I came back from my first assignment to Baghdad in late 2003. We were living in Jakarta. Harry had just turned one. I'd been gone nearly two months. Harry wasn't sure who I was. He clung to Mary. Rather than reconnect with Harry, I pulled strings with head office to return to Iraq.

Mary and I met Belle the same day we first saw Patrick. She was twelve months old. We hadn't intended to adopt two children, but when Mary and Belle locked eyes, that sealed it. We couldn't adopt Patrick and Belle together because they weren't related. It took two years navigating Indonesian bureaucracy to get Belle out of the orphanage. Because Belle was born with a cleft palate, we were told to 'choose' another child. Orphanage officials seemed embarrassed about her appearance. Mary wouldn't be swayed, even when told to stop visiting Belle.

Unlike Patrick, who quickly settled into home life, Belle struggled. She was virtually deaf because of ear infections caused by her cleft palate. She didn't speak and had mostly been confined to a cot with no toys. Those Mary brought always disappeared. Orphanage staff saw Belle as a nuisance, particularly at night when she howled from pain in her ears. Food leaked from her nose because of a large fistula on the roof of her mouth, essentially a hole in her poorly repaired palate, which had been operated on at a local training hospital. Early on when Mary asked why Belle made no attempt to speak – she used hand gestures – she was told, 'Oh, she's just lazy.' Occasionally, Belle was isolated in a small room with no windows. We weren't allowed to pay for any surgery until a Jakarta court ratified her adoption.

Belle was almost three when her ear canals were cleared. The Indonesian surgeon wasn't optimistic she'd hear properly. But she did. The first time Belle heard music she literally stopped in her tracks. It must have been magical for her. To this day Belle's Airpods are always either in her ears or nearby. Once she could hear, she began speaking. She'd spent long enough imprisoned in a soundless world. She propelled herself into life and her spirit soared.

But Belle struggled to make friends at kindergarten in Jakarta and beyond. Inclusion can be out of reach for children who look and sound different. Mary took Belle to Australia but failed to convince a cleft palate team to operate. There was a schedule for such surgeries. Belle would have to wait her turn.

Eventually, in 2007 in Jerusalem, Mary approached a surgeon originally from Texas who wore a cowboy hat and boots. He lamented the psychological trauma Belle must have endured having to wait. He and another surgeon repaired Belle's palate as best they could. A small fistula remained, but food no longer dripped from Belle's nose. Belle began speech therapy. She was a brave and determined child and she learned enthusiastically.

Even so, every night for years Belle would wake, screaming in terror, writhing on her bed. We held her tight to try to comfort her. Our beautiful daughter was diagnosed with PTSD at the end of 2019 from abuse and neglect she suffered in that pitiless orphanage.

*

I haven't spared Belle, either. A couple of years ago Mary and I were watching TV one night at home in Evandale when Harry rushed in, saying he could smell smoke. In our long hallway, I smelt it too. Belle, thirteen at the time, was sitting cross-legged on the floor of her bedroom, unwashed clothes strewn about. She held dead matches in her hands.

'Do you have any idea of the danger you've put us in?' I roared at her. 'You could have burnt the house down.'

I towered over her tiny frame, then stormed back into the living room. Mary was furious with me. Harry had disappeared. I went back to Belle's room and yelled some more. She was too shocked to cry.

I've yet to tell Belle I'm sorry. *What sort of father am I?*

—

In bed, I stare into space. Inert. All I see is fog. Then I see Saeed Chmagh lying on a waist-high stone slab. The photograph shows two men preparing Saeed's body for burial. They wash his face with water. Saeed's left foot, gouged off by the Apache's cannon shells, is on the slab, next to his mangled leg. A small, wet orange towel covers Saeed's torso. Other parts of his body are wounded by shrapnel, but they look smooth compared to the grotesqueness of his left leg and severed foot.

I must have pushed the deaths of Namir and Saeed into the deepest recesses of my mind because they were the last of my traumatic memories to surface when I unravelled. I realised this a month ago when Mary mentioned how we first heard about the Collateral Murder tape two days after Julian Assange shocked the world with the footage. I can't recall why Mary brought up the video but what she said stopped me cold. I'd virtually forgotten that day in Devonport when I'd seen the newspaper article about the tape. Until that moment last month, I'd kept Namir and Saeed at arm's length even as I was losing my mind. I would use their names but without emotion.

I ordered my first book about PTSD after Mary reminded me about the tape. That same day – 25 June 2016 – I decided to start a journal, maybe because of the overwhelming thoughts competing for space in my muddled brain. Sitting in front of my laptop, typing words on a page, cleared a bit of the haze.

But I could no longer ignore the fast approaching ninth anniversary of Namir and Saeed's deaths on 12 July. It was time to open an email folder marked 'Namir and Saeed', a black hole I hadn't been into in years. It was time to try to understand why guilt and shame had begun to seep into every pore of my skin, every cell of my body, splintering my heart and my soul.

So much is coming back, creeping into my consciousness.

I lost my staff.

I scrutinised the contents of the email folder for weeks: a report by the Reuters pictures team showing a Google Earth map of Namir and Saeed's rough movements on the day they were killed; a catalogue of every frame from Namir's two cameras; my notes from the off-the-record briefing the two generals gave me on the military's so-called investigation into their deaths; the transcript from the Crazy Horse 1–8 crew.

What I couldn't do – what I've never done – is watch the full Collateral Murder tape. Those first few minutes the generals showed me was all I could take.

The emails, documents and photographs made me understand that I'd failed to protect Namir and Saeed. And I was a coward for not confronting the Reuters leadership when they accepted the US narrative that the military investigation into their deaths was thorough, the rules of engagement followed, no attempt made to cover up what happened. All lies. Reuters let the matter quietly drop despite outrage around the world and inside the company over Collateral Murder. This opened the way for history to blame Namir for the bloodshed. My memory is so warped that I, too, believe it. I know more about what happened to Namir and Saeed than probably anyone alive, yet I've stayed silent for nearly a decade. Mute. Me, the journalist. I'm unworthy of the Iraqi national flag my staff signed and gave to me when I left Baghdad.

I decided to ask numerous Iraqi and foreign colleagues what they thought of my actions, or lack of them. They were either in Baghdad with me at the time or had worked there. Part of me wanted condemnation. The other sought validation. Please understand how I feel, I begged silently. They all defended me, tried to make me feel better. It was war, they said.

That made it worse. *No one understands me.*

I barely understand myself. I use the words guilt and shame interchangeably, unsure how they differ. I don't know that, on top of PTSD, I'm suffering from a condition called moral injury.

'You've become your own judge, jury and executioner,' Mary told me. In a sense she is right. But I have to reckon with myself. Find the truth.

While I immersed myself in that email folder, Mary found a therapy program for journalists run by the Traumatic Stress Clinic in Sydney, with sessions delivered by Skype. The director was a renowned expert who, in a radio interview Mary found online, said journalists suffering from work-related trauma were not getting the help they needed. She urged me to listen to it.

I'm not sure why I did. Maybe it was the look Mary gave me when I donned tradie earmuffs after she turned on the TV to watch a political affairs program. A raised voice triggers me. I had to do something.

But the Traumatic Stress Clinic told me it would take five to six months to get in. I put my phone on the small coffee table Mary bought in Jerusalem's Old City. My head dropped.

How am I going to recover?

I tried to bluff the kids. Don't worry, I said. But they knew.

'I'm one brain snap away from a *ledakan*,' I wrote in my journal that day, using the Indonesian word for 'explosion'; I was worried Mary, who doesn't speak the language, would freak out if she saw it. She freaked anyway when I sent a text message hours later that said: 'Thank you for loving me babe'. She thought I was saying goodbye.

———

From bed I can faintly hear my closest friend, Jeremy Wagstaff, tapping away on his keyboard in my study next door. Jeremy, who is British, flew down from Singapore two weeks ago to support me. He also works for Reuters. Tall and thin, Jeremy can impersonate the Queen of England and every character from *Dad's Army*. My kids think he's the funniest person they've ever met. But neither his charm nor his concern over my welfare has had any impact on the bosses. Not long after my 'one brain-snap from an explosion' moment, a month ago, Jeremy sat down with them in Singapore. He explained how dire my mental health was, gave them copies of WhatsApp messages he'd exchanged with Mary with her permission. The bosses kept the notes but told Jeremy they couldn't deal with him because he wasn't family.

They were bureaucratic and cold. It was like he'd dragged them away from more important matters. 'We can't be having this conversation,' one said. They never contacted Mary and told Jeremy to pay for his flight to Tasmania and either work while at my home or use annual leave.

After seeing for himself how sick I was, Jeremy went over the heads of the Asia bosses and rang New York. More silence.

I don't think to call out to Jeremy. What would I say? I understand now why people take their own lives, if it means peace, an end to the exhaustion, the pain.

I've had vague sensations of not wanting to live since my PTSD diagnosis. In bed right now, I want to die. I'm a burden to my family. 'Toxic' is the word I use to describe my presence in the house. Numb and withdrawn one moment, unpredictable and enraged the next. *Mary and the kids will be better off without me.* My brain is too confused and heavy to see a future for myself. I can't live with the pain of being alive any longer. I just crave peace.

The South Esk River will do the job. Over the past two months Tasmania has suffered its biggest floods in a century. One night the South Esk rose so fast it swept away thousands of livestock. The south-western approach road to Evandale and a bridge across the river disappeared. From our living room, the South Esk was an ocean under a grey, moody sky. The roar echoed up to our yard for weeks. The South Esk is still a seething mass of water this evening, contemptuous of its banks.

Now, in the darkness of the bedroom, I visualise the river. Rain and melted snow drive the current hard. I shed my clothes at the bank. I walk in, bracing against the frigid water. I let myself fall face first, opening my mouth to the muddy torrent. The river takes me. Done. Relief.

*

36

I lie still. Eyes open. Not sure for how long. I'm crossing a point of no return. Breaking some taboo. I roll out of bed like an old man. I'm in the same track pants, T-shirt and socks I've worn for days. The hallway is dark and quiet. Patrick, Belle and Harry are probably in their rooms. Their doors are shut.

I sit on the couch in the living room, staring at the floor. Mary sits beside me, her arm across my shoulders.

'I'm toxic to my family. I want to walk into the river and find peace,' I say. 'I just want to be alone.'

Mary is gentle but firm: 'You need to be hospitalised in a psych ward, and soon.' She had been waiting for this moment.

'Isn't that a bit drastic?'

'No, you've hit rock bottom.'

Jeremy comes out. He must have heard me on the creaky floorboards in the hallway. Mary tells him what's going on.

'Mate, Mary is right. You need to be hospitalised.'

'What would the kids think?'

'It will help them too if you get intensive treatment,' Mary says.

I remember little else except going back to bed. Mary and Jeremy debate whether to take me to the emergency department at Launceston General Hospital or call an ambulance. They decide I should stay home, where they can watch over me. Trying to get me to emergency might push me over the edge.

That's what I recall from this conversation. It's what I wrote in my journal the following day. I locked on the starkest words because I wanted evidence the fault was mine.

'You need to be hospitalised in a psych ward, and soon.' Yes, Mary said that, but I don't recall the loving context because I felt undeserving. It might have been easier for my family if I'd come home from Iraq with a physical wound. Something they could see. Patrick, Belle and Harry struggled to comprehend my anger, unpredictability and silence. It was like a secret they had to carry outside the house. It wasn't as if the family made a rule. The children just didn't know how to talk about me. If I missed an event, Mary or the children said I was sick. When the kids had parties at home, I stayed in bed to avoid the noise.

Mary was a wall, a barricade between me and the children. Ever hypervigilant, she helped them tiptoe around me, trying not to drop cutlery, slam a door, clang dishes in the sink or have the TV too loud. She believed I'd get better. She researched treatments even though I protested for years that I was fine. But she always had one hand on the door.

Mary had two red lines: violence against her and allowing my trauma to seriously damage the kids. She was determined to protect them. Mary stood on two fronts – with me, and with Patrick, Belle and Harry. She'd look at small houses in Evandale when driving through the village, wondering if she could afford any alone. As a young journalist in Tasmania, she reported the trials of men who murdered their female partners. She would soon work in a women's shelter, and counsel refugees from Afghanistan and Africa who had experienced family violence.

Mary explained PTSD to the kids, told them why my eyes were puffy in the morning. They knew I'd worked in dangerous places overseas. That I had trouble sleeping, sometimes had nightmares. Above all, Mary reassured Patrick, Belle and Harry that I loved them, wasn't angry with them. That as a family we'd get through this.

3

Do I really need to be here?

Captain Morgan rum and Panadol usually help me fall asleep. Not tonight. Not before being admitted to the Ward 17 psych unit. I slip out of bed and walk down the hall. Red embers glow from the living room wood heater. I add a few logs. The fire warms me. The house is still. Darkness lies beyond the windows.

I turn on the TV and watch *Fury*, a movie about a fictional American tank crew fighting behind enemy lines in Germany in 1945. Brad Pitt plays Don 'Wardaddy' Collier, a haunted tank commander. I've seen *Fury* before. The exhaustion in Collier and his men draws me back. Their leaden eyes are mine. Their vacant stares. Tanks, trucks, jeeps and boots churn the earth into mud. I drink a last rum and coke in the early hours and go back to bed, sleeping fitfully.

I see dead eyes in the bathroom mirror the next morning. When did I last smile? I'm not sure Ward 17 will help.

*

Mary drives me to Launceston airport for my flight to Melbourne. We hug, say goodbye. I show no emotion. Mary keeps hers in.

Mist rises off the craggy Ben Lomond mountain range to the east, visible through the large windows of the departure lounge. My right foot taps the floor. What if the doctors at Ward 17 reject my PTSD diagnosis? Or say my symptoms are minor? What if they try therapy that doesn't work? My stomach knots. I want to be admitted. I want to get better. Mary is sure Ward 17 will be the start of my recovery. I hope she's right.

Journal entry. Launceston Airport. Aug 11, 2016: I am bad for my family and sometimes my family feels bad for me. I hate to say this, but I can't wait to get a private room, feel peace and quiet for the first time in how many years? When have I had the chance to feel this? No chaos. No meals to cook, no unexpected visitors, no stress of the dog barking. How shameful is it to even think this?

Will I emerge healthier, wiser? More in control? I HAVE to, for the sake of my family.

It's been two weeks since I thought about killing myself. Mary sat next to me when I called my psychiatrist the following morning and said we both believed I needed hospitalisation. Mary insisted I go interstate given the lack of options in Tasmania. My psychiatrist sounded a bit surprised but referred me to Ward 17, a specialist PTSD facility formally known as the Psychological Trauma Recovery Service at the Heidelberg Repatriation Hospital in Melbourne. It treats veterans, first responders, other survivors of traumatic workplace injury and victims of crime. My warzone exposure meant I'd fit in, he said.

The trickiest issue was the roughly $800 daily fee. My private health insurance didn't cover Ward 17 and the intake officer said they avoided self-funded admissions because it put too much pressure on patients and staff to get quick results. I'd have to ask Reuters, but would they care? I procrastinated for a couple of days then emailed the bosses:

I fear I am not far away from a total breakdown. Sometimes I find it hard to make it through the day without drinking, sometimes I struggle to get out of bed. My kids are suffering, with two of them not wanting to go to school and avoiding other activities. Mary my wife is training for a new line of work but has not been able to give it her full attention because of my condition . . . I spoke to one of the [Ward 17] intake officers yesterday, who said the usual length of stay was 2–4 weeks . . . Is this something Reuters could fund? I'm obviously not expecting an immediate answer, as this is a lot of money. I'm happy to discuss on the phone.

I didn't mention my suicidal thoughts. Jeremy Wagstaff had just flown back to Singapore and worked behind the scenes, lobbying as many as six bosses and getting paperwork together. Four days after I sent my email, I got a brief reply to say Reuters would pay. No one called.

Instead, my former Baghdad colleagues rallied around me, welcomed me back into my community, my tribe. Self-isolation had been one of my biggest enemies. The day after I was suicidal, I'd emailed Andrew Marshall, a Cambridge University educated Scot who had left Reuters five years earlier. I first worked with Andrew in Jakarta during upheaval in Indonesia in the late 1990s. A few years younger than me, I'd envied Andrew's meteoric rise in Reuters. He was the company's first bureau chief in Iraq after the US-led invasion in March 2003. Two Reuters journalists were killed while Andrew ran the Baghdad operation.

Andrew broke mentally before I did. He knew I'd follow, but I never let him near me emotionally when we worked together.

'I'm in a bad way,' I wrote to Andrew, who lives in Edinburgh. 'At the top of the causes of my PTSD is guilt over Namir and Saeed, from their deaths to the way I handled everything afterwards, including when the video was released.'

Andrew replied: 'I've wanted to speak to you for so long, because I felt sure you were in a dark place after Iraq, just as all of us have been, but I realised I would have to wait until you were ready to discuss things in your own time . . . There is so much to say, but maybe the most important is that you are not alone. Nobody who went through what we did came out the other side unchanged and undamaged.'

Andrew's warmth and empathy lifted me. I could see beyond the blackness. And the prospect of getting answers at Ward 17 – for a moment I thought this might be a turning point. That I could get my life back on track and spare my family more pain.

In another email soon after, Andrew talked about moral injury, something I'd never heard of.

'From what I understand of PTSD, people are affected in various ways. One of the most toxic, which frankly goes beyond PTSD into more mysterious and even spiritual territory . . . is "moral injury," which seems to be connected, but is not well understood,' he wrote.

The first item to appear when I googled moral injury was a series called 'A Warrior's Moral Dilemma' by American war correspondent David Wood, published in the *Huffington Post* in 2014. American veterans were mired in moral and ethical ambiguities from Iraq and Afghanistan, Wood said: shooting a child; losing a beloved comrade; feeling betrayed when a buddy was hurt because command made a bad decision; surviving a road-side blast that killed others; seeing evil done and being unable, or unwilling, to intervene.

'It is what experts are coming to identify as a moral injury: the pain that results from damage to a person's moral foundation,' wrote Wood, who had covered American soldiers in combat for 35 years. 'Moral injury is a violation of what each of us considers right or wrong . . . a bruise on the soul, akin to grief or sorrow, with lasting impact on the individuals and on their families.'

Wood quoted those experts in his series, the tiny number of clinicians treating American veterans for moral injury. It didn't take long to find their pioneering research and definition of potentially morally injurious experiences: perpetrating, failing to prevent, bearing witness to, or learning about acts that deeply transgressed someone's moral and ethical values.

Bingo.

I'd failed to prevent Namir and Saeed's deaths.

Moral injury's signature symptoms were guilt and shame. Again, that was me. There was an overlap in symptoms with PTSD such as anger, depression and anxiety. Sufferers of both self-medicated with alcohol and drugs and sometimes took their own lives.

It felt a bit weird applying a condition seen in veterans to myself because I hadn't been a soldier. Sure, I'd spent time in Iraq, but I was never shot at or witnessed combat. Mortars and rockets flew over the Reuters compound, headed for the Green Zone. That's why I call myself a correspondent who covered war; I'm always embarrassed when referred to as a war correspondent. I see a distinction. But I knew I was onto something with moral injury.

Journal entry. Launceston Airport. Aug 11, 2016: Moral injury. Feel this describes me. Namir and Saeed. Maybe the key is to come to some sort of acceptance and then seek atonement. How does one atone for nine years of guilt? If I can get beyond moral injury, what next? What else is lurking there? There must be more under the surface from Iraq, Aceh and Bali.

———

The Launceston departure lounge is busy. I sit where I can see everyone. I'm jumpy and don't want any surprises. People stare at their smartphones. What are they thinking? How many are normal? What is it like to feel normal?

On the plane, I return to the morning after Islamic militants bombed two nightclubs in Kuta Beach in 2002, killing 202 people, including 88 Australians. That was the first time I saw what a bomb could do to a human being.

In my head, I see the rotting corpses in Indonesia's Aceh province after the Boxing Day tsunami in 2004. Lying by the roadside, tangled with debris under bridges and in canals. About to be shovelled into mass graves by earthmoving equipment.

One day I watched two men drag the decomposing body of a girl from rubble and twisted trees before lowering her into a small grave dug with a farm hoe. She looked about ten. She might have been clothed. I can't remember. It was just over a month after the tsunami swept away the town of Leupung, home to as many as 10,000 people. With few shovels, gloves or masks, several dozen men had been burying the dead. They had thousands more to dig out, they told me. Not a single house or building remained standing. Men carried purple body bags to a large, freshly dug hole. They placed the bags in the hole, then emptied them – so the dead would decompose quicker, one man said. Heads and torsos tumbled out. Another man placed the heads side by side in the grave, as if to give them a semblance of dignity. The smell didn't seem to bother the men. I walked away and called my boss on my satellite phone. I've got a story for today, I said. *'Shocked Aceh town, utterly destroyed, buries its own.'*

Mostly, however, I think about Namir and Saeed.

Lost in my thoughts, I forget to wear earphones after getting into a taxi at Melbourne airport. Music calms me: Linkin Park, Coldplay, Sia, Pink Floyd. The taxi crosses a bridge. Its tyres on the grooves sound like the rotors of a Black Hawk helicopter: suddenly I'm in Baghdad. Noise and heat bounce off the concrete as Black Hawks, always in pairs, land and take off. My muscles tense, my heart skips a beat. There is too much of everything in Melbourne. Too many cars, too many traffic lights, too many buildings, too many houses. When did everything get so loud? I'm hot, claustrophobic. The earphones stay in my bag. My mind is elsewhere.

The taxi stops outside the Heidelberg Repatriation Hospital. I go to a security post and get directions to Ward 17.

Pulling two suitcases, I walk past a garden of stone monuments and plaques honouring the sacrifice Australians have made in a century of war. The hospital opened in 1941 as a military facility. It now serves the wider community, but still treats veterans and war widows. I turn left at the Flanders Wing, breathing in the smell of soggy vegetables. Patient food is being cooked nearby. On my left is a weatherboard building shaped like a military barracks. It looks shuttered, the blue paint faded long ago. That's the old Ward 17, a Vietnam veteran called Ray Watson will tell me in a couple of days. Veterans suffering psychological wounds who served in World War Two, the Korean War and the Vietnam War slept four to a room. Ray was one of them.

The new Ward 17 is a little further on in the Coral-Balmoral Building, past the Diggers Way road sign. The grey, flat-roofed building was named after Australia's largest battle of the Vietnam War. Veterans of that conflict still feel the pain of indifference of successive governments. Belated recognition of their service. A society that never understood them and still doesn't.

I stop at the glass door to Ward 17.

I've been frightened before, like getting lost in the Iraqi city of Falluja in late 2003. While it was dangerous to travel anywhere in Iraq, Reuters foreign journalists still did. One exception was Falluja, a Sunni insurgent stronghold 60 kilometres from Baghdad, just off the highway. It was the end of my first assignment to Baghdad, and Andrew Marshall and I were being driven to Amman, Jordan, when we saw that US troops had blocked the way. It looked like there had been an attack up ahead. All traffic was being diverted into Falluja, home to 250,000 people.

'Get as low as you can,' said a bald Irish bodyguard in the front passenger seat, gripping an AK-47, as mud-coloured buildings drew closer.

I squeezed my body into the space behind the driver. Andrew did the same behind the Irishman. A blanket was thrown over us. Breathe slowly, I said to myself. My ears became my eyes. I listened for noise that didn't belong: gunfire. Shouting. Sudden braking or acceleration. Our driver had never been to Falluja, the Irishman mumbled. Fuck. We turned right. Then left. Right. Left. Eventually, after 45 minutes, the driver got back to the highway, beyond the American roadblock.

A few months later, insurgents ambushed a convoy of vehicles in Falluja, killing four American security contractors. They hanged two of the beaten and charred bodies from a bridge.

Standing outside Ward 17 is a different kind of fear. I'm about to cross a line, be admitted to a psych ward. I don't know anyone who has spent time in one. They've kept it quiet if so. I walk in. On my immediate left is a nurse's station encased in sound-proof glass. Four or five staff in casual clothes are talking or writing up notes. No one notices me. Ahead and off to the right is a common room with comfortable couches around an old wooden coffee table and a dining area of laminated tables and plastic chairs. Bearded men wearing track pants, T-shirts and flip-flops move in slow motion. I'm wearing a chocolate-coloured fleece pullover, new blue jeans and the R.M. Williams boots Patrick tried to walk in as a toddler. Bloody overdressed for a psych ward. I knock on a window and a small, smiling woman opens it.

'I'm being admitted today,' I say, hoping no one will hear me.

The woman has my paperwork. She fastens a red plastic band around my wrist that gives my name, date of birth, home address and hospital number. The process takes a few minutes but feels like an eternity.

Journal entry. Ward 17, Melbourne. Aug 11, 2016: Do I really need to be here? Am I this bad?

A nurse in her early twenties takes me past the dining area and couches. The men are lined up at a counter, waiting for lunch to be served. They are big and intimidating, their arms covered in tattoos. Veterans, I reckon. I want to hide. I don't belong here. I'm not worthy. I bet those blokes saw real action, earned their place, fought on a frontline. I think of Reuters journalists who've spent far more time covering war and natural disasters than me and yet are still working.

We turn right into a wide corridor and enter Room 11. There is a large window on the door with shutters fixed on the outside. The bed is a hospital one on wheels covered by a thin faded quilt. The room has a long built-in desk, plenty of space for my laptop, notepads and books on PTSD, war and trauma.

'Do you have any medication or sharp things?' the nurse asks.

She takes my antidepressants, Panadol, razors, nail clippers and antifungal cream. I have an itchy arse. Stress makes me itch. Three nurses will have asked what the cream is for by the end of the day. Ward 17 is no place for embarrassment.

I glance around the room as the nurse rummages through my suitcases for prohibited items such as alcohol. There are green buttons to press for assistance on the cream-coloured walls. Red buttons for an emergency. The door handles slope down at 45-degree angles to prevent patients hanging themselves. Staff sometimes do random breath tests, the nurse says. No more Captain Morgan, I think ruefully. A large window looks out onto tall gum trees. In the distance, beyond the hospital grounds, I see a Returned and Services League club. They sell alcohol and cheap meals. I later hear that RSL employees watch for anyone wearing a hospital wrist band. My bathroom is big enough to fit a wheelchair. No towel racks. No gap between the hand-rail next to the toilet and the wall.

The nurse gives me questionnaires to complete and wants to do some medical tests. But have lunch first, she says.

The dining area is the last place I want to be, but I swap the jeans and boots for track pants and worn joggers, my usual attire. About seven or eight men are eating silently together. One of the kitchen staff gives me a bowl of soup. I sit at an empty table, avoiding eye contact with the men. I haven't thought about this moment. Do I introduce myself? What will patients think when they know I'm a journalist? Will they be suspicious? Think I

48

don't belong here? I'm not sure I do. The men keep to themselves while I try to suppress the anxiety in my chest.

—

Later, I fill out the questionnaires. My goals for admission, I write, are:

- *Stop being numb, especially with Mary.*
- *Learn to cope with family life.*
- *Find the old husband and father I used to be.*

Next is a standard checklist for PTSD, which first appeared in the benchmark of modern psychiatry, the US *Diagnostic and Statistical Manual of Mental Disorders 3 (DSM-3)*, in 1980. That came after years of lobbying by the US Vietnam Veterans Against the War organisation, and by psychiatrists who treated soldiers traumatised by the conflict.

The American Psychiatric Association, publisher of the *DSM* (now *DSM-5*), says PTSD can occur from exposure to actual or threatened death, severe injury or sexual violence. This might involve living through the event; witnessing it happen to others; learning a family member or close friend has suffered trauma; or being repeatedly exposed to trauma like first responders. PTSD can result from a single event or an accumulation of experiences.

The four main clusters of symptoms are:

1. Re-experiencing: Reliving trauma through distressing and intrusive thoughts and memories. These can take the form of flashbacks and nightmares.
2. Avoidance: Avoiding anything connected to the trauma,

such as people, places and situations. Thoughts and conversations can be impacted; what you read and watch.

3. Mood: Negative changes in thoughts and mood, such as emotional numbness to loved ones, depression, isolating yourself, unable to enjoy things, feeling detached from people.

4. Arousal: Anxiety, irritability, getting startled easily, hypervigilance, rage, difficulty sleeping and concentrating, and reckless behaviour.

I've come to Ward 17 expecting to meet soldiers, coppers, ambos and firefighters. But I have no idea PTSD reaches into virtually every occupation. I'll meet a schoolteacher, a truck driver, a chef. I don't know yet that scores of journalists I worked with in Iraq and elsewhere are struggling with mental illness. I'll find out later that most stay quiet for fear of losing their jobs. I'm also largely ignorant of PTSD's prevalence among survivors of childhood sexual abuse, rape and domestic violence and in marginalised communities.

A twenty-question PTSD checklist asks me to rank my symptoms in the past month using a scale where 0 is 'not at all' while 4 is 'extremely'.

- Repeated, disturbing and unwanted memories. 4.
- Feeling jumpy or easily startled. 4.
- Blaming yourself or someone else for stressful experiences or what happened after. 4.
- Having strong negative feelings such as fear, horror, anger, guilt or shame. 4.
- Feeling distant or cut off from people. 4.

A Hospital Anxiety and Depression Scale asks how I've felt in the past month. I note that I feel tense or wound up 'most of the time'; worrying thoughts go through my mind 'a great deal of time'; and I look forward with enjoyment to things 'hardly at all'.

On another questionnaire I write that I'm bothered by headaches, tightness in my chest, shortness of breath, feeling tired, low energy, loose bowels and trouble sleeping.

Another document asks me to complete the following statement: 'When I'm angry or upset please DON'T make me feel even worse by saying . . .'

I fill in the rest.

'. . . that when you are unhappy the whole family is unhappy'.

This is directed at Mary. I know she is being truthful when she tells me this, but I resent her for it.

The nurse returns. We walk to the medical treatment room. I sit in a green chair with long arm rests, trying to relax. The nurse takes my blood pressure, heart rate and temperature. She asks about my symptoms. Then:

'Have you had suicidal thoughts?'

Where did that come from?

After processing what she said for a few seconds, I tell her about the South Esk River.

'I just craved peace,' I say.

'Are you suicidal now?'

Again, she catches me off-guard.

'No,' I reply firmly.

There is too much on my mind. I'm jumpy and exhausted.

'Do you need Valium?'

'No. I've never taken Valium.' That would be weakness, I think to myself.

Next I do a 90-minute interview with a psychiatry registrar in a patient–therapist meeting room. Background first: born in country New South Wales to working-class parents. Studied economics at Sydney University. Decided to become a journalist after climbing the Berlin Wall in 1990 while backpacking through Europe. Started work for Reuters in Jakarta in 1993.

Mary and I agreed to start a family while living in Jakarta in mid-2001, I tell the registrar. At 37 and having worked non-stop for nearly twenty years, Mary was burnt out. She didn't get pregnant initially, so we settled on adopting. Both Mary and I have younger sisters who were adopted, and she had already decided when we lived in Vietnam in the late 1990s that she wanted to adopt. She wanted to enable a child, not save them. One story she did for Reuters TV was about a teenage boy from a central Vietnam village who'd been born with no arms below his elbows and no legs beyond his thighs. His father, a former South Vietnamese soldier, had mixed the ingredients of the Agent Orange defoliant the Americans dropped on vast swathes of jungle. The boy wanted to go to university, so he saved money to get the bus to Ho Chi Minh City, formerly Saigon, to enrol. Told he had to pay an enrolment fee, he went home and saved that money too. Still, the university wouldn't let him sit the entrance exam. Maybe they were embarrassed: he was a stark reminder of the war. Undeterred, this young man sat outside a lecture room and took notes, having made a contraption so he could write. Eventually, the teachers let him sit the exam, believing he'd fail. He passed and became the university's second disabled student (the first was his sister). He played soccer, did his share of cooking and cleaning at his student accommodation. Mary watched in disbelief as he rode a modified pushbike through Ho Chi Minh City's peak-hour traffic.

In late 2001 we adopted Patrick. Mary got pregnant a few months later with Harry. We brought Belle home in mid-2003.

Many people have often said Patrick and Belle were fortunate to be adopted by us. No. We were blessed they came into our lives.

At Ward 17 with the psych registrar, I rattle off my exposure to trauma – Bali, Aceh and multiple assignments to Iraq. There are other bombings and earthquakes, my year-long posting to Jerusalem, but I stick to the Big Three, focusing particularly on Namir and Saeed.

'I need to get on top of my guilt and shame,' I say. 'There is no point telling me to be rational. I know I could have done more for Namir and Saeed. How do I get beyond this? Have I got moral injury?'

The registrar doesn't offer much in the way of answers. She is doing a case history, asking questions, taking notes. My right foot taps non-stop. I fidget. My cheeks are flushed. I'm coherent but edgy. I speak tremulously, she writes.

Concerned about my agitation, the registrar asks the nurses to check on me every hour.

'It's just a precaution,' she says, but I know what it means.

My afternoon nurse is a man born in Lebanon. In my room, we talk about the Middle East. I search my past for Arabic words. One phrase comes back easily: *wayn alainfijar?* Translation: where was the explosion?

At dinner, I sit alone. Half a dozen men and women chat at the next table. A burly, bearded man announces he can smell coconut. I freeze. The smell comes from the expensive moisturiser on my hands: Desert Essence Coconut Hand and Body Lotion. I try anything to stop the itching between my fingers. The smell is the focus of his attention, and now the table. I've only just arrived, and I don't know that some smells can trigger people with PTSD. It's not like the burly man seems agitated, but he's hellbent on finding the source. He asks the kitchen staff if it's the food. I keep eating. About ten minutes later the man is making a cup of tea near the kitchen. *Bloody hell, he's still talking about the smell.* I go over, look him in the eye, and say I have coconut moisturiser on my hands.

'I knew it,' he says, whirling around to men near him. I scurry off.

Ward 17 is quiet, apart from the radio-static tinnitus in my ears. I noticed it ten to fifteen years ago. The ringing gets louder when I lie down or am stressed. Still, I feel a bit calmer. Being in a psych ward is strange. But as the hours have ticked by, any lingering denial about where I am can't compete with the cream-coloured walls of Room 11, the green and red buttons, and my bed on wheels.

Today has been so busy I've yet to call Mary. When I do, we talk about my day.

'I want to find that old husband and father,' I say.

'The new one will be good, wise and understanding,' Mary says.

Near the end of our chat, after Mary talks about the kids, I note how peaceful Ward 17 is, an unintentional criticism of home life.

'Things feel good here tonight,' Mary says, in the process expressing her true feelings. 'No unpredictability, no ripple effect.'

Fuck. I really am toxic. If I don't recover, I might need to move out. Give the family a break.

I tell Mary I need to go to bed.

We'd agreed before I left to be honest about our feelings even if it hurt. Our marriage needed this to heal. Ward 17 would give us the safe space to do so. Problem was, I'd forgotten the conversation. Maybe I had too much on my mind. Mary recalls taking a deep breath before saying those words, but she miscalculated, as she later put it. It was too soon.

To love someone with PTSD can be like reaching for the unreachable, Mary will tell me. Being met day after day with a wall of emotional numbness or a squall of anger, with silence and the fear that any sudden noise you make could evoke memories of a mortar attack. But you stick it out. You shield the children, keep the family together, she will say with unflinching honesty. Other days, she says, you just want to run, to breathe, away from the unpredictability.

It will take me a long time to understand this. For years, Mary had filtered the full impact my trauma had on her and the kids. Tonight, my first in Ward 17, they could relax, knowing I was at one of Australia's top inpatient mental health facilities. At this point, Mary never believed our marriage would disintegrate, but she knew it was deeply fractured. I was too numb to see the strain it was under.

I ease between well-washed sheets and pull blankets and the thin quilt over me. No need for alcohol; my brain has had enough for one day. I drift off but wake half a dozen times during the night. It's okay, I say to myself. It's your first night in a psych ward.

I'll be like this for the next five weeks, even on sleeping tablets. The shutters opening and closing on my door window wake me sometimes. I see the outline of a face, a nurse doing hourly checks. Still, my narrow bed and worn quilt is comforting. I feel safe.

But that doesn't stop the nightmares.

4

An angel from Tehran

'No unpredictability, no ripple effect.'

The words hang over me when I wake the next morning around 6.30 am. It's the truth. I'm a shocker to have around.

I push those thoughts aside and soak up the silence and simplicity of my spartan room. I'd love to stay under the covers, but before being admitted I'd vowed to walk each morning.

The outside temperature on my phone shows it's a bit warmer than Evandale but still beanie weather. I throw off the blankets and old quilt, get dressed and move quietly through the empty corridors. I ask at the nurse's station if I can go for a walk. Ward 17 is not a locked-down facility but there are restrictions on going out, especially in a patient's first week. A nurse checks my file. A walk is fine. I sign out.

With British band Coldplay pulsing in my earphones, I retrace my steps from when I arrived. The Heidelberg Repatriation Hospital is big, nine entrances off four streets. Easy to get lost. I spot a gravel path after leaving the grounds and walk briskly through parkland, a children's play area and then the leafy suburb of Ivanhoe until I see a narrow footbridge. Ducks are paddling in a creek below. I stop and watch. I'll do the same walk nearly every morning until I'm discharged.

Back at Ward 17, I sign in, shower and eat breakfast in the dining area before other patients show up. Nurses refer to me as 'low profile' in their notes during my first two days.

I'm reading in my room when someone knocks on the door. A well-dressed woman wearing oval-shaped glasses smiles and introduces herself as Dr Maryam, my psychiatrist. As we walk to a patient–therapist room, I ask Maryam – all staff go by their first name – if she is Arab. She's Iranian, or Persian as she puts it. I grimace. Iranians don't like being called Arabs. Different language for starters. Maryam laughs. The psychiatry registrar and nurse from the previous day are waiting. I sit in a chair against the wall. Maryam has pale skin and long black hair parted in the middle. Her face radiates intelligence and kindness. Speaking with a slight accent, Maryam tells me she was born in Tehran. She was a toddler when Ayatollah Khomeini made a triumphant return from exile in 1979. The Islamic Republic of Iran was proclaimed soon after. She was in the Iranian capital when an earthquake killed more than 31,000 people in the ancient city of Bam in 2003 and helped with aid efforts there.

Maryam, 40, has walked in my world. I sense she is also curious about me. Maryam has read the notes from the registrar and nurse but wants to hear me tell my story, starting with my career. This is routine for me now. I pluck dates, places and death tolls from memory. Maryam writes down every event.

I stop after about twenty minutes; time to let Maryam speak. Maryam thanks me for sharing and gets straight to the point.

'Dean, I feel like I've been listening to a journalist reporting a story,' she says, leaning forward a little, a soft smile on her face.

The wheels in my head begin to turn.

'That was how you spoke about your career, like you were referring to someone else,' Maryam says. 'The level of detail was one giveaway. You're intellectualising your trauma, showing little emotion. Compartmentalising your experiences, avoiding dealing with them.'

I don't surprise easily – why would you when you're numb to the world? But my brain, my gut, tells me Maryam is onto something.

I lean forward. 'What do you mean, intellectualising my trauma?'

'You are in your journalist's skin,' says Maryam. 'You are trying to tell *a* story, rather than tell *your* story. It's less painful that way.'

Journalist's skin. Maryam has seen straight through my mask. Reuters covers news wherever it breaks around the world, whatever the topic. I was the perfect fit from the moment I joined as a stockmarket reporter in Jakarta in 1993, getting sent to cover an earthquake on Sumatra three months later that killed 200 people. I wasn't an investigative reporter who spent months burrowing into the underbelly of politics and business, or a features writer with elegant prose. I was a methodical news agency journalist who did one story after another, with energy and stamina that amazed the bosses. There was never time to process anything. There was always another story to do, more questions to ask, coverage to plan, staffing issues to sort out.

I loved it.

'Avoidance is a natural defence mechanism,' Maryam says. 'But it won't help you confront your trauma. Treatment starts by acknowledging what happened.'

I lean back, more relaxed, tilting my head to one side.

'When talking about the Boxing Day tsunami, you held back tears,' Maryam says. 'Why?'

'I instinctively suppressed the emotion,' I reply. 'That's who I am.'

I take Maryam into the Baiturrahman Grand Mosque in the centre of Banda Aceh. The earthquake at 7.58 am local time had a magnitude of 9.1, the third biggest ever recorded. Its shallow epicentre was 150 kilometres (94 miles) off Aceh's coast. The massive undersea convulsion pushed waves as far as East Africa. US government estimates put waves that crashed into Aceh's coastline at up to 30 metres (100 feet) high. People had no warning.

I walked by corpses rotting under a burning sun on debris-filled streets to get to the mosque three days after the tsunami. Doors, window frames, mattresses, fridges, cars and bodies clogged the normally grassed area at the front. The mosque itself was remarkably unscathed. I went inside, past white pillars and stained-glassed windows. Bloated bodies, most still clothed, lay in rows on marble floors. The smell had concussive force. Dazed survivors, covering their noses with cloth or their hands, walked numbly past each body. Presumably trying to find loved ones. I counted every contorted, blackened corpse until I got to 158. Someone later gave me a handkerchief to wrap around my face. How could I truly convey the horror?

'I still see those bodies,' I tell Maryam.

'Why did you count them?' she asks.

'A news report needs specific details, numbers,' I reply. But it was more than that.

'I felt compelled, like someone had to do it. They deserved to be counted.'

I tell Maryam about a child who often intrudes into my thoughts. I was at Banda Aceh airport about ten days after the tsunami to cover a visit by Colin Powell, then US secretary of state. While waiting for Powell to speak to the media, I walked around the airport. Injured Acehnese were still being evacuated to better equipped hospitals. Some were in tents on grass, away from the runway. I saw a young girl whose face had been burned, probably in a fire triggered by the earthquake. She lay on a stretcher, her head on a pink pillow. She looked like Patrick. Before I could ask aid workers about her, tears filled my eyes. I had to walk away.

Five years later, while searching the Reuters pictures data-base for a photograph to illustrate a story I was writing about Indonesia, the child's face appeared. I was instantly confused and disoriented. I read the caption. An Indonesian colleague had taken her photograph that day. Her brown eyes stared at the camera, at me. Hands in surgical gloves gently put ointment on the dark scabs and pink fleshy wounds across her tiny face.

'I've only cried a few times,' I say to Maryam. 'What sort of person shows so little emotion despite what I've seen? There must be something wrong with me.'

'You became very good at compartmentalising things,' Maryam says. 'At avoiding troubling memories.'

There is a pause in our conversation. I change the subject to Namir and Saeed, saying I need to deal with my guilt and shame over their deaths. Everyone says I shouldn't blame myself. Everyone wants to make me feel better. No one understands. I need to watch the WikiLeaks video while I'm here.

What I don't say, but what I mean, is that watching Namir and Saeed die might force me to cry.

'You're not ready for the tape,' Maryam replies firmly, before herself changing the subject.

'How are things at home?' she asks.

I tell her what Mary said about the 'no ripple effect' with me in Ward 17.

'How do you feel about that?'

I shrug. 'It hurts, sure, but I know I'm toxic to my family.'

There is something you need to know, I say to Maryam, who already has my basic family background. It's a secret I've kept for a decade. Never told anyone. But something about Ward 17, the 24 hours I've been here and now this connection I feel with Maryam has made me realise she needs the full story. Understand who I really am.

I lean forward, elbows on both knees. Head down, right foot tapping.

In early 2006, Mary and I were preparing to leave Jakarta for Jerusalem. My entire focus was the new job, it was a big promotion. I was going to fly to Jerusalem and find a house while Mary took the kids to stay with her parents in Devonport for two months. They would then join me. One evening, several weeks before we left Indonesia, Mary told me she was pregnant. She was in her early 40s, the pregnancy unplanned. Patrick and Belle were five, Harry three.

Mary was both nervous and joyful. I was furious, having never agreed to a fourth child. We'd talked about it, but I felt it would be too expensive to have four children, even though Reuters paid school fees and housing for someone of my seniority.

I told Mary to have an abortion. Mary was shocked. She and the children would stay in Tasmania, she said. You go to Jerusalem. What Mary meant was that she'd leave me and have the baby.

'I felt a rupturing in our marriage, but I stuck to my position

61

because I thought I knew what was best for our family,' I say to Maryam. 'My coldness was astonishing.'

Mary had had an abortion seven years earlier, when we lived in Vietnam in the late 1990s. We wanted to have a family at some point, but not then. Mary had dreamed of being a foreign correspondent since her early teens and her TV career with Reuters had taken off. She was travelling constantly. Mary was passionate about the people she reported on, they were living in conflict and poverty, the aftermath of war. She admired their courage and resilience and was determined to bring their stories into living rooms around the world. Mary chose to terminate that pregnancy, with my full support. Nevertheless, she wrestled with her decision for many years.

We didn't have a conversation about her 2006 pregnancy. We've barely talked about it since. But something about Ward 17 has made me realise Mary must carry a deep wound. I worked the phones that night in Jakarta to arrange an abortion as soon as possible. Eventually, I got her an appointment in Perth. She would travel alone, and that would be that.

Mary didn't need the appointment because she miscarried that night.

—

Maryam and I are near the end of our session. She confirms my PTSD diagnosis, a result of cumulative traumatic events. The Bali bombings, three assignments to Iraq from 2003 to 2004 and the Boxing Day tsunami 'softened' me up before Namir and Saeed were killed while I was Baghdad bureau chief from 2007 to 2008, Maryam says.

Besides PTSD, she tells me I have major depressive disorder, another name for clinical depression. She will change my anti-depressants because the ones I'm on don't seem to help, and she prescribes a drug for my nightmares, which will either stop them or make them harder to recall.

We're finished. My feet have tapped the floor for two hours. They must have noticed, but neither Maryam, the registrar nor the young nurse said anything. Exhaustion washes over me. I thank Maryam, who says she will see me again early next week. The nurse wants to take my vital signs. In the medical room, I apologise for keeping her so long.

'No, it was fascinating, you've had such an interesting career,' she says.

I think to myself, 'Yeah, and now I'm paying the price.'

Journal Entry. Ward 17, Melbourne. Aug 12, 2016: Why did Mary marry me if I am so numb, so emotionally cold? How does one deal with all this emotionally? Do you just cry? Atone? Something about the last 24 hours has made me realise I am mentally ill. I hadn't realised the extent of it before. I'm sick. Have been for a long time . . . I have a right to be here. I feel that now.

Later that afternoon I feel comfortable enough to explore the rectangular-shaped Ward 17. A couple of doors along is Ray Watson, the Vietnam veteran. His door is wide open. Ray lies on his bed watching a movie on a portable television he must have brought from home. He doesn't notice me.

Opposite our corridor is a small internal courtyard with fake grass, two exercise bikes and a big barbecue. In a corner room is a TV, couches and books. A few patient rooms form the end of the rectangle, then on the other side is a laundry, two interview rooms, the medical room and a larger TV space. A couple of men are watching something. They don't notice me either. In the common room and dining area, someone has started a word game on a whiteboard. The schedule of weekly group sessions is pinned up. Newspapers are spread over the old wooden coffee table, where patients have used pencils to scratch messages or sign their names and dates of admission.

'A lot of the work of getting better is done at this table. Sit down. Relax, talk and get better,' says one message.

'People who judge you by your past, don't belong in your present,' reads another.

Maybe I will be accepted in Ward 17.

5

Eggshells

I'm eating breakfast alone on my second morning in Ward 17, a Saturday, when Ray Watson shuffles in.

'These lazy coppers. Still in bed,' Ray says to no one in particular. He then looks at me: 'You're not a copper, are you?'

I shake my head. I've never been mistaken for a police officer, although Ray might be pulling my leg. I don't say I'm a journalist. Ray sits diagonally across from me. I know he's a Vietnam veteran because of the T-shirt and cap I saw him wearing the day before.

I ask Ray about his deployment. Within minutes Ray points to the three places on his ageing overweight body where he was hit by bullets in 1966. After leaving the military he was a policeman and a country firefighter in Victoria. A lifetime of trauma exposure. He's been to Ward 17 many times.

'My fucking problem is I can't stop living in 1966,' he says.

That was 50 years ago! Will that be me?

Ray wanders off and a younger man sits down for breakfast,

directly opposite. His name is Brett Lewindon. Brett was in the Royal Australian Infantry Corps for eight years, serving in East Timor twice, 1999–2000 and 2003, which he says fucked him up. Brett then joined Victoria Police. This is his first admission and his police bosses don't know he's here.

My eyes widen. 'How is that possible?' I ask

'I told them I had a physical illness and needed time off. DVA [Department of Veterans' Affairs] is paying for my treatment. If my police sergeants know I'm here, they'll sack me,' he says.

I sit back. Brett hasn't made a big deal of his predicament. He seems resigned to a fate he has no control over. There is an integrity about Brett, who looks in his late 30s, six foot tall. He's wearing blue jeans, hiking boots and a red and black checked lumber jacket.

His last police call out before coming to Ward 17 was cutting down a 21-year-old man who'd hanged himself in his garden shed. Before that, it was the death of a three-week-old infant, suspected to be SIDS (sudden infant death syndrome) that turned out to be homicide. Both parents were methamphetamine users.

I ask him what sort of help you get from the police force.

'The senior officer does a debrief: *You okay mate. Yeah, all good.* That's it. You can't admit you're fucked.'

Brett never tells his wife what he sees. Domestic violence cases are tough when babies are there. Crying babies trigger him most. Brett has one child and another on the way.

'Young coppers have no idea what they're getting themselves into,' he says.

A few weeks later, with the help of a police union official, Brett will tell his superiors that he's in Ward 17 and can't return to work.

*

I haven't come to Ward 17 to interview my fellow patients. But now I'm genuinely curious. What happened to them? Can they still do their jobs?

Brett is my first exposure to the fear – apart from my own – that stops people disclosing a mental illness to their bosses. Fear they will be judged. Fear of losing their job. I'll meet scores of men and women in Ward 17 who feel deeply betrayed because their organisations didn't support them when they developed PTSD. Veterans, coppers and paramedics who were forced out, told they couldn't serve their country or their community. First responders tossed into a workers' compensation system that doesn't just worsen their mental health but destroys it. Destroys their chance of recovery. Destroys their relationships.

Employers, workplace regulators and governments are fully aware of the cabal of insurers, lawyers and so-called independent psychiatrists who prey on mentally injured police and emergency service workers. They know about the emotional and financial abuse, the systemic denial of benefits, how insurers hire investigators to spy on people to accuse them of being frauds. How claims are drawn out for years until first responders give up or take their own lives.

DVA is little better, as the 2022 interim report by the Royal Commission into Defence and Veteran Suicide showed. What the royal commission has yet to address is why the government of former prime minister Scott Morrison chose not to follow up landmark independent research that identified hundreds of suicidal veterans who left the military from 2010 to 2014; effectively buried the same research after it showed alarming rates of mental illness among a veteran cohort of nearly 25,000; and shut down a major research project into new and more effective ways to treat soldiers and veterans suffering PTSD and other mental illnesses. Those extraordinarily callous moves, which the mainstream media missed, have condemned our servicemen and women to decades of poorer mental health outcomes.

After breakfast, I put in my earphones and walk to a bookshop in Ivanhoe. I'm hoping to find *Man's Search for Meaning* by Viktor Frankl. Maryam had thought it might interest me. I'd never heard of the book or Frankl but was intrigued. An Austrian Jew who lived in Vienna, Frankl was a well-known psychiatrist at the outbreak of World War Two. He survived three years in Nazi concentration camps, including Auschwitz. To my delight, the shop has a copy of a slim book Frankl wrote in nine days after being freed at the end of World War Two.

Man's Search for Meaning is grim. Frankl paints a graphic picture of beatings, humiliation, slave labour and near starvation rations. But it's clear in the opening pages that Frankl wants to show how people can find meaning in even the most appalling circumstances.

'A man who becomes conscious of the responsibility he bears toward a human being who affectionately waits for him, or to an unfinished work, will never be able to throw away his life. He knows the "why" for his existence, and will be able to bear almost any "how",' Frankl writes.

There were three main ways to find meaning, he said. The first was to create a work or do a deed. The second was loving another person. The most important was to rise above a hopeless situation, to turn personal tragedy or unavoidable suffering into triumph.

I sit back in my green hospital armchair, feet on the bed and think for a few minutes. I can find meaning in life by raising awareness of PTSD. I can tell my story and by extension help people who have no voice. Just three days here and I have a sense of purpose. Hope, even. Given I was suicidal less than three weeks ago, it's a momentous shift.

That's not to say I'm cured. But it's easier to get out of bed when you have meaning in life. Finding meaning becomes my compass.

Late on Sunday afternoon, I hear patients returning from home leave. Most patients live in Melbourne or country Victoria and spend the weekend with family or friends. I muster the courage to go to dinner. Ward 17 is nearly full. I line up at the kitchen counter, get my meal and join a table with Ray. I sit next to a skinny guy with stubble on his gaunt face. He looks early 40s and is covered in tattoos. Within seconds I accidentally drop my fork on the table. The skinny guy jumps out of his chair.

'Fuck, sorry, mate,' I say. 'I know what it's like.'

First the hand moisturiser, now this. At least it's a conversation starter.

Sean Callaghan tells me he's a veteran and clearly sensitive to unexpected noise. Sean says he's been barred from a pub near his flat for raging at staff when they throw empty bottles into a skip bin off the first floor around ten o'clock each night. The table discusses how to solve the problem.

Eventually, his arms crossed, Ray comes up with a solution: 'Napalm.'

Journal entry. Ward 17, Melbourne. Aug 14, 2016. I see these guys and think fuck, this could be me for years. Haggard. In and out of places like this. Constantly on meds. What do I have to do to get myself better? I have to be honest in saying that I enjoy the peace and quiet. Not tripping over shit on the ground in the house, not cooking meals, just responsible for myself. Would I be better off on my own? Would my family be better off without me? Maybe I need to rent a little place near Evandale so I can see Mary and the kids regularly. Can't believe I'm saying this. Must talk to Maryam about it.

—

The following morning, I attend my first group session. I stay in my room until the last moment. I want to get to know people, but I'm still unsure of my place. I walk into the meeting room adjacent to the common area. Patients are sitting in chairs arranged around small tables pushed together. I nod at Ray, Brett and Sean. I introduce myself to half a dozen other patients, all men. Some chat, they seem to know each other. There is a small pool table in the corner behind a whiteboard; art and drawing materials in boxes on a side bench. The room has a few small windows. It's a large, private space. A young occupational therapist is running the session, which is about sensory modulation.

'Who has issues with sensory overload?' the OT, who I'm going to call Michelle, asks.

All the men do. They start chipping in: sirens, alarms, bright lights, noisy children, aggressive people, crowded anything – shopping centres, train stations, supermarkets, cafes. Soldier J, a veteran who served in Afghanistan, says his kids, five and eight, know they need to be quiet to avoid 'setting him off'. He won't go outside his home in rural Victoria in case anyone sees him. Sean says his wife and son wait with trepidation each morning to assess his mood.

Michelle suggests using noise-cancelling headphones at a train station or supermarket. She talks about strategies such as dim lighting at home, playing soft music, taking hot showers, and squeezing a stress ball. Modify your sensory environment where possible, she says.

Some comments have already been a bit ribald when Michelle mentions relaxation massages, which is the cue for laughter and bawdiness. 'Your wife will be bloody suspicious if you tell her you're going for a massage,' one veteran says. 'I hear a happy ending costs fifty bucks up the road,' adds another. Michelle, in her mid-twenties, gets the conversation back on track with intelligence and tolerance. She seems used to it.

One patient then uses 'eggshells' to describe his impact on home life. The tone changes instantly. Others nod. I'm not contributing, just listening. But I can't believe it. These blokes are like me.

Back in early June, I'd just got home from a trip to the Tarkine rainforest. I'd been on sick leave for three months. I found solitude and peace among the ancient trees of the Tarkine, a 450,000-hectare wonderland in Tasmania's north-west. Trying to recognise myrtle from leatherwood, celery top pine from blackwood. I placed my palms and body against tree trunks. Skin on bark. I lost myself in the rough of the myrtles. The smooth of the sassafras with their saw-tooth edged leaves. I marvelled at colourful fungi and lichen, cool to the touch. I kayaked along the glassy surface of tannin-stained rivers, mist rising off the mountains in the distance. On this trip I'd slept in a wood cabin built by miners in the 1930s. For three nights I didn't have a single nightmare. All I heard was the crackle of a wood fire and the gurgle of Fraser Creek. I embraced the challenge of finding my way among poorly marked tracks. Then I returned to the big house on the hill overlooking the South Esk River, to a family that loved me but feared my unpredictability. In turn, I feared theirs.

'The children and I are tired of walking on eggshells,' Mary said as my backpack and muddy boots lay on the living room floor. An unexpected arrival of Harry's mates had set me off.

Eggshells!

Something in my head snapped. Mary and I were standing near the large glass doors in the living room that open to the backyard. I paced like a caged animal, waving my arms in the air.

'Aren't I making progress?' I shouted at Mary. It was a ludicrous question. I was getting worse. Mary had never seen me like that.

'Don't *ever* use that word in this house again!' I boomed.

Mary walked out of the room without looking at me or saying anything, convinced I would hit her if she challenged me further.

I've little memory of that outburst. I just believed that if your loved ones were walking on eggshells, you were no good to them, and I couldn't face that.

The blokes in Ward 17 hate the word eggshells too, but agree it describes life for their partners and children. I sense the same guilt and shame in them about the pain they cause at home. Their stories validate mine. I like the honesty. One patient says he thought of taking an overdose last week. I'm starting to belong.

6

An 'introduction' to treatment?!

I was given an information pack when I arrived at Ward 17. It included a booklet that outlined the topics covered in group sessions as well as a one-page note called 'Treatment of Post-Traumatic Stress Disorder (PTSD): The Linen Cupboard Metaphor'. The note showed two linen cupboards. In one, everything was neatly folded. The other was a mess.

For someone with PTSD, distressing memories are like items in the messy cupboard, the note explained. Brush past, the door flies open, things fall out. The standard response is to shove everything back in and slam the door. In other words, don't deal with them. Avoidance. But the distressing memories – often intrusive images or flashbacks – stay jammed and jumbled in the cupboard, and the door can swing open at the slightest touch. Things you don't want to relive but which can be triggered by something you see, hear, smell or touch.

The note on the linen cupboard metaphor said treatment for PTSD involved slowly taking things out, examining them carefully, folding them neatly, and putting them back on the right shelf. This way, traumatic memories have their proper place. You can find them if you choose to. But they won't come back uninvited so often.

I loved the simplicity of the message and stuck the note on a whiteboard above my desk.

I'm in a good rhythm by the start of my second week at Ward 17. I get up each morning about 6.30 am. Go for a walk. Attend one or two group sessions run by the OT, Michelle. Maybe meet with Maryam or Christina Sim, the social worker. Eat three meals. Read, write, reflect, sleep.

While I'm feeling more comfortable, I do continue to tap my feet in group settings, in one-on-one sessions or in the dining room. When I write or read in my room, they are still.

I'm making progress. But a word I keep hearing near the nurse's station and in the common room puts me on edge.

Discharge.

While no one has mentioned the prospect to me, I tell the nurses I don't want to talk about discharge. I'm petrified about going home. I'm not here for knee surgery. I'm fucked up, can't live in the real world. I still think about the South Esk River, although my thoughts are not as strong as the night I wanted to walk into its wild waters.

Each Friday, Michelle puts out a roster of group sessions and activities for the following week. The sessions cover understanding PTSD and treatment options; managing anger; dealing with anxiety; coping with depression; improving communication with spouses/partners; and making sense of our journey, finding meaning in life. There are groups with less heavy content such as healthy cooking, art and music therapy and reflexology.

Each group runs for 45 minutes. Michelle schedules three a day from Monday to Thursday, as well as a gym or hydrotherapy session each afternoon at a veterans' complex next door. Nothing is compulsory. Friday is usually left free for patients who want to go home for the weekend.

Michelle's role is to show us how to live better with PTSD. She is part educator and part coach. She wants us to understand our triggers so we can manage our symptoms and find new ways of doing things. She works with a maturity and confidence that belies her age. Everyone respects her knowledge and passion.

One sunny winter's afternoon, Michelle takes us to practise mindfulness among 521 small white wooden crosses planted in green grass on the hospital grounds. The crosses represent the souls of Australians who died in the Vietnam War. My body sinks into the cool grass. Michelle's voice blocks out the hospital bustle as she asks us to focus on our toes, then feet, ankles and all the way to our heads. I think of those soldiers, some barely old enough to be men.

Not everything goes to plan, but Michelle has the temperament to cope. While preparing the meeting room one day, she accidentally bumps into the pool table. One of its foldable legs collapses and the table crashes to the floor. Michelle looks at several of us standing just inside the room, laughing. We saw it happen.

'Would you believe it's not the first time I've done that?' she says with relief, knowing we could have hit the ceiling.

During one session, sirens sound from a fire station at the corner of the hospital grounds. A female copper catches my eye. Others nod. Michelle doesn't hear the sirens and expresses surprise later when asked. It's the same when a helicopter passes overhead during another meeting. People with PTSD hear the world differently.

*

One morning I sit with Michelle and tell her I can't stick to a routine. Gone is the news leader who left nothing to chance, planning coverage of set-piece events, who carved his personal future into blocks, knew what he'd be doing in five years.

'I used to be so organised. Now, I'm useless,' I say.

Michelle encourages me to draw up a weekly schedule. Don't worry if you miss a day, she says. She shows me an app called Rain Rain Rain to help me relax, and suggests I get noise-cancelling headphones. I download the app and use it every night and sometimes during the day when I rest under my faded quilt. When I later give Michelle the sheet of paper with almost every waking hour covered with a task, she ticks me off.

'You need time to take it easy, do nothing!' she says.

With so much to absorb, I'm often exhausted by mid-afternoon. It's a battle of wills with the nurses to steal a nap. They want us awake during the day so we sleep at night. I put a note on my door in the afternoon that says 'meditating'. They soon wise up. I try one that says: 'I'm sleeping, only wake if you're Dr M'. They ignore that too.

I bond with other patients in group sessions and at meals. At breakfast I usually say 'Morning', not 'How are you?' Most patients, me included, look crap: bags under eyes, vacant stare, slow shuffle to the mobile meds station manned by two nurses. By my count there are five coppers, three old soldiers and several younger ones, two prison guards and a truck driver. The trauma we experienced on the job creates an instant connection. I don't have to explain myself. My new friends get it.

Hearing their stories validates mine. They have nightmares, flashbacks, anger and anxiety too. Each of us has damaged a relationship with a partner, some beyond repair. We share our vulnerabilities and inner fears as well as our hope that there might be a better future outside the quiet predictability of Ward 17. We laugh in group sessions, at the dining table or sitting on the couches around the old coffee table. Black humour is a way of dealing with heavy subjects. Not a single patient says, 'Quiet, there's a journalist in the room.'

Soldier J is a beefy good-natured veteran in his early 30s who did three deployments to Afghanistan over four years. He has a ginger beard and military tattoos on his arms and shoulders. He also has a black PTSD assistance dog called Benny. One evening, Soldier J explains how the border collie/blue heeler cross senses his emotions. Sitting on the couch, Soldier J pretends to cry. Benny jumps up and licks his face, pawing at Soldier J's chest until he focuses on the dog. In a crowded supermarket, if Soldier J gets stressed, Benny will lead him to a quiet place. If Soldier J is depressed and won't get out of bed, Benny barks, not loudly, just enough to motivate him to move. At breakfast in Ward 17, Benny works the tables, knowing someone will slip him a piece of bacon. In the evenings, when the strict unit manager has gone home, Soldier J takes Benny's PTSD coat off. We throw his ball up the long corridors. Benny scampers off and ambles back, always eager for more.

Standing in the corridor near my room one night, Benny at his feet, Soldier J says he was 21 when he joined the army as a parachute rigger. It's a highly skilled role in which soldiers inspect, repair and repack parachutes as well as jump themselves. Soldier J tells me one day an IED exploded in an Afghan town, wounding some kids. Soldier J had photographs of the kids put up to show those who supported the Taliban what was being done to civilians. The Taliban raided the hospital and killed the kids in their beds. Soldier J blamed himself.

'That's what fucked me up. I feel so much guilt,' he says.

The ground moves beneath me. Soldier J's story is among the most horrendous I've ever heard. *How will he recover from this?* Australians have no idea what our soldiers are trying to cope with. And I get where he's coming from. The moral responsibility he feels. I keep my journalist mask on and let Soldier J talk. I've got no answers, no advice. He isn't looking for any. And I'm pretty sure he doesn't want me to say, 'Don't blame yourself.' Instead I say, 'That's a fucked-up situation mate.'

Solid at 80 kilograms in the army, Soldier J is now 130 kilos, on his third admission and another round of electroconvulsive therapy (ECT). ECT is used for severe depression that hasn't responded to other treatment. Patients get a muscle relaxant and general anaesthetic before an electric current is passed through the brain to induce seizures that relieve symptoms. Mental health charity SANE Australia says roughly eight in ten people experience dramatic improvements. Most have some short-term memory loss, which often gets better with time.

Sean Callaghan was in the army for fourteen years. He's a few years younger than me. He had a safe upbringing, went to good schools, never went without. In 1995, a fellow soldier was blown up in front of him on a training exercise in Southeast Asia. The man had jumped into a small trench to throw a grenade but accidentally pulled the pin on a second one attached to his belt. Sean survived, left the army in 2005, and then got lost.

'For me it was, what do I do? Where do I line up? What's my routine?' he says.

Sean has taken crystal meth every day for five years. He's been off it for four weeks. He ignores the street sellers when he goes out to buy cigarettes: 'You chasin mate?' they say.

Sean's sunken cheeks, darting eyes and jerky movements give him away.

Sean is always good humoured, fun to talk to. On a group walk to a coffee shop he gets into a hospital laundry cart and starts it up. He wants to stay clean and tackle his PTSD. He has a new sim card to avoid contact with people who might lead him back to drugs. Sean wants to get a diploma to work in drug awareness and education, speak at schools, maybe get into counselling. One evening, Sean shows me how easy it is to buy ice off the internet. There are photos everywhere. We realise three coppers are sitting with us. We all laugh.

———

In my first group session on anger management, I blow up. The lack of empathy from my Reuters editors has broken me, I say. I'm red-faced, arms waving. I got one phone call two days before my admission. That was it. Others say their bosses haven't called in more than a year. What is it about PTSD that makes it so hard for bosses to pick up the phone? The consensus is we're seen as damaged goods.

Some coppers use the word 'contagion' to describe their experience: it was like they had a contagious disease. Their bosses, even colleagues, wanted nothing to do with them (I learn years later that the workers' comp process encourages isolation of the injured employee). As a result, they lost their identity, their sense of self. Other patients say that once they put their hand up about their mental illness, they were fast-tracked for discharge (vets) or dismissal (coppers). *Will I ever work again*, is a question that haunts just about every patient except the Vietnam veterans who are in their 70s.

What we have in common is rage towards our current or former employers. A deep betrayal that binds us together.

At least I have a job. In late June, I worked up the courage to ask the bosses if I could train and mentor young reporters in Asia when I got better because I couldn't do news anymore. My psychiatrist in Hobart had said I wouldn't recover unless I did something different. What was once second nature filled me with dread, I wrote in a lengthy email proposing the new role. I attached a note in which my psychiatrist said I might never do journalism again because of the stress. I was terrified my proposal would be rejected.

A few days later, the Asia boss greenlit my proposal in a brief email. I could start slowly, maybe writing one or two blogs a month on the topic of my choice, with no pressure on deadline. A part of me was relieved. I also seethed that no one called. I'd been off work at that stage for four months. Reuters kept paying my salary and didn't question the sick leave I was taking. But no one from Singapore or New York tried to understand my situation, open a conversation about my treatment or future.

Didn't they get how sick I was? I felt so alone. I'd detached myself from my family. My self-esteem and confidence had disintegrated. I lived in a fog, felt worthless.

One morning a week into my admission, I wake about 4 am with a headache. I get up an hour later and go for my walk. I quicken the pace along the gravel path, striding faster and faster in the darkness, fists clenched. My blood burns at the indifference shown to me by Reuters. The 23 years I've given to the company. Saying yes to tough assignments. The sacrifices my family have made. I get to the creek. There is a tunnel for walkers on the other side. I go through. I want someone to mug me. I'll kill them. I crave physical violence.

Journal entry. Ward 17, Melbourne. Aug 23, 2016: Here's my question, has Reuters worsened my PTSD?

I'll think about this often in the years ahead, concluding that the most critical factor in trauma recovery is the quality of someone's support network: family, friends, GP, counsellor, psychologist/psychiatrist, employer, workmates, access to hospital services, housing, the justice system. Yes, a support network extends beyond family and friends. It's the breadth and depth of those networks and how they function together – not the original trauma – that largely determines recovery outcomes. In other words, whether a trauma survivor can find safety. Process their trauma, rebuild relationships, find purpose in life, and live with dignity. Sure, all of us in Ward 17 – soldier, copper, paramedic, firefighter, journalist – knew what we were getting into. What we never signed up for was betrayal and abandonment.

The biggest barrier to my recovery will be Reuters. I'll discover this is another form of moral injury and that healing from organisational betrayal will be harder than overcoming the many ways I failed Namir Noor-Eldeen and Saeed Chmagh.

I start writing my first blog under the new training and mentoring role. I call it: *Reporter's Notebook: PTSD, My Toughest Story.* I open with the ways I thought of killing myself, then explore my confusion as my symptoms worsened until I entered Ward 17. I show it to Maryam, who sees it as work and says I'm not ready. I want to raise awareness of PTSD within Reuters given how I've been treated, I say. I plan a second blog about my admission and a third on my recovery plan. I've given no thought to what Patrick, Belle and Harry will think. They don't know I've been suicidal. They might not see the story, but what if it goes public? Maryam understands my motives and says I'm well qualified to get the message out. But I shouldn't rush into publishing. I need time to process.

'Viktor Frankl's book has had a profound effect on me,' I say. 'I once had meaning in life covering big stories, running large operations and doing things for my staff.'

'Don't be impatient. Your mind is moving too fast trying to understand and deal with this. It won't happen overnight,' Maryam replies.

I've ignored Maryam on the amount of reading and writing I'm doing. My gut tells me I'm on the right track there. The old Dean, the 'man of action', as my friend Jeremy Wagstaff called me the other day, is back. But Maryam says I'm using the blog to avoid the work of processing my memories and unfreezing my emotions. I need to think about this.

Maryam then says my admission is an 'introduction' to treatment. She is reinforcing a point she has made every session, that my journey will be long, don't expect an 'aha moment'. This is something I haven't absorbed nor noted in my journal. Maybe my brain blocked what it didn't want to hear. But Maryam's use of the word 'introduction' cuts through me like Mary did with 'eggshells', though I react differently. I stare at Maryam, shocked. A sense of doom curdles in my stomach. I thought I'd walk out of here cured. A new man.

'Many things are starting to surface that need to be dealt with,' Maryam says softly, sensing I've been rocked. 'You are in crisis.'

I'm ready to reveal everything to my treating team, but not to be told Ward 17 is simply an introduction to treatment. That means recovery will take years.

7

Panic attack

Back in my room, I sit at my desk, both legs pumping like pistons. I should rest, think about what Maryam has said. But I've got an appointment this afternoon with Cait McMahon, Asia-Pacific managing director for the Dart Center for Journalism and Trauma, at her office near Royal Melbourne Hospital in Carlton. The Dart Center is based at Columbia University in New York. It promotes informed and ethical news reporting on violence, conflict and tragedy. It also educates journalists about trauma and mental health risks. Cait is a psychologist who has explored the links between journalism and trauma since the mid-1980s. I want to ask her about trauma among Australian journalists.

I catch a taxi to Carlton, a busy suburb near the CBD. I haven't told Maryam about the appointment because I'd get an earful.

In a cafe, Cait expresses no surprise I'm in Ward 17. Moral injury is becoming a major component of trauma among journalists, she says, validating how I feel about Namir and Saeed.

Cait talks about extensive research she has done on Australian journalists. She has discovered some have become caught in an 'existential dilemma' of not knowing how to respond when covering human suffering.

'Journalists have said to me: "I didn't know whether I should act as a journalist or a person in a certain situation." What they were saying was: "Should I be objective and detached and observe, or should I get in there and do something?"'

'The person who chose to respond as a journalist and the person who was quite clear in responding as a person had reasonably low post-trauma reactions. The ones who were confused about their role were the ones with the highest post-trauma reactions.'

Towards the end of our conversation, Cait asks if I've heard of a former photographer for *The Age* newspaper who developed PTSD after doing a series of stories with relatives of Australian victims of the Bali bombings to mark the first anniversary of the attacks. I hadn't. Cait says the award-winning photographer has the worst PTSD she has ever seen. The photographer sued Victoria's leading broadsheet for breaching its responsibility to care for her mental health when *The Age* sacked her in 2008 after she was off sick for more than two years.

The photographer used the acronym AZ to protect her identity in the trial, the first of its kind in the world for a journalist. The Supreme Court of Victoria ruled against AZ in 2013.

I'm outraged. How can a major employer like *The Age* – then part of Fairfax Media, now owned by Nine Entertainment – treat someone like that? I feel a kinship with AZ and offer to visit her. 'That's kind, but you need to focus on your own recovery,' says Cait, who gave evidence on behalf of AZ. She refuses to give me AZ's name or contact details.

My 90-minute chat with Cait motivates me. The Dart Center might be another avenue to spread awareness of PTSD within the journalistic community. But it's time to go back to Ward 17.

Cait worries about me finding a taxi. I'll be fine, I say. She insists on accompanying me across the road, then advises me to head towards Royal Melbourne Hospital. As I walk, the buildings on either side close in. They look alien. Ugly. Menacing. My heart races. I can't see any taxis. I need to cross another road to reach the hospital. The traffic light stays red for what feels like forever. My feet tap the ground. People next to me must sense my agitation. Green! I rush across but can't find the entrance or exit to the hospital. It's 4 pm, peak hour is starting. What if I can't get a taxi? What if it rains? Maybe I can call Ward 17 and get them to send one. Maybe I can check into a hotel to get off the streets. Where are the hotels? *What is happening?*

Suddenly, an empty taxi appears and stops. I jump in, slump against the back seat, close my eyes. I've forgotten Michelle's breathing strategies. My heart and head pound.

Back at Ward 17, my sanctuary, I want to hug the nurses. One offers me Valium when I say I freaked out.

'I don't want to become dependent on meds,' I say.

She comes to my room: 'You are sick, you are in hospital. Take the meds, don't deny you had a bad panic attack.'

I give in. Drowsiness washes over me.

—

I stay in my room for the next couple of days, sleeping and reading. I skip group sessions, only emerging for meals. Michelle comes in and gently says it's been noticed I'm isolating myself. The nurses say my treating team are worried. One nurse asks how I'm feeling. 'Having a mental health day,' I reply.

When do you get to a point where life feels okay? When do you feel you're functioning reasonably normally?

I realise how much work I've got ahead.

After a few days, I join a cooking group run by the Ward 17 dietician. We make tortillas. It's relaxing and the tortillas are delicious. Mary and I agree it's best to park the blog while I'm in Ward 17. It's distracting me like Maryam said. I get back to group meetings.

In my next session with Maryam, I say the panic attack terrified me.

'I've thought about whether this will affect me when I travel. What if I go somewhere new? How much planning will I need to do? Is this my future?'

Maryam says the panic attack could have stemmed from reliving things with Cait outside the safe Ward 17 environment. I was also amped up after our chat, I add. Maryam smiles when I say I'm shelving the blog. I'd obsessed over it. She nods, pleased I've used the O word. I'm not sure why – maybe because I'd written about it in the blog – but I ask Maryam if I'd exaggerated my suicidal thoughts. I don't want to seem like an imposter.

'There was no garnish there,' she says. 'I think you were looking for a way out, right?'

'Yes. I wanted to feel peace. I wanted to escape the pain, the fog. The guilt. The numbness.'

'Do you feel suicidal now?'

'No, because I have a mission, to fight for those who have PTSD. And to reconnect with my family.'

Maryam tells me to take time out over the next few days to relax, watch TV.

I do a brain shift that I know will exasperate Maryam.

'I can't. I feel like I'm in the middle of a big story – this one is PTSD – that needs to be told. I'm like a reporter racing to the scene of a disaster. I want to publish so I can raise awareness, help others.'

I'm leaning forward in my chair, adrenaline pumping through my body.

I tell Maryam about offering to see AZ.

Maryam gets that look in her eyes.

'This is exactly what I mean,' she says. 'Focus on your recovery first and stop trying to help others. That's probably your guilt making you want to do that. Get yourself well first. You need to slow down. All this reading, you're like a med student studying for an exam. Buy a book that has nothing to do with PTSD and war.'

'But I've found my calling.'

'That's fine, but don't rush it. Frankl didn't write his book until he was out of the concentration camp.'

I talk later to my mate Jeremy Wagstaff on WhatsApp. Maryam says I'm overdoing it, I tell him.

'I think she's right, but I can't help it,' I say. 'She wants me to read a book that has nothing to do with war or PTSD.' I can't find anything that interests me, I tell Jeremy, so I went back to reading *Trauma and Recovery: The Aftermath of Violence – From Domestic Abuse to Political Terror* by American psychiatrist Judith Herman. 'What do these shrinks know anyway?'

'She has a point, mate, that's not exactly light reading,' Jeremy replies.

*

Journalism's greatest lure is offering a ringside seat to the action as history unfolds. The trade-off was to stay detached. This combination exacted a price – denying emotions that others might have expressed.

But journalism is also guiding my approach to recovery. Maryam and my treating team want me to take recovery nice and easy. I want to wrestle my demons into submission like a journalist would, throw the kitchen sink at them. What book haven't I read? Who else can I speak to? I'm trying to control the knowledge of PTSD, the illness. I embody that third person Maryam referred to, watching from a distance. A major challenge will be learning how to open myself up emotionally and sit with whatever uncomfortable feelings emerge, rather than pushing them away.

8

Sex

I'm reading in my room late one afternoon during my first week in Ward 17 when I hear loud footsteps approaching then a firm knock. It's Christina Sim, the social worker. Christina is Malaysian-Chinese, with straight dark hair down to her waist. She shakes my hand with a big smile, looking at me kindly through large prescription glasses, a thick folder of notes in her left arm. Christina asks if we can talk in my room.

When I filled out the paperwork on my first day, I wasn't sure what to make of the social work partnership document. I expected to see psychiatrists, psychologists and nurses at Ward 17. Not a social worker, an OT, a dietician and a spiritual care worker. I soon learned that Ward 17 has a range of experts because PTSD is a complex illness. This multi-disciplinary approach to treatment is overseen by a psychiatrist, in my case Maryam. My team discuss my progress once a week and can access each other's notes.

Christina's role is to focus on my relationships at home, she tells me. She has helped people with PTSD for nearly 30 years.

As with Maryam, I immediately like Christina.

She asks about my symptoms. Emotionally, I'm shut down, I never cry, I say. But I'm also unpredictable, super sensitive to noise. If something sets me off, I get angry or agitated. I can't cope with the chaos of family life. Mary and the kids would be better off if I was dead, and so would I. End the pain.

Where these words have come from, I don't know. I haven't spoken so darkly to anyone in Ward 17.

'This is the beginning of your recovery,' Christina says quietly, leaning forward in the green chair I use at my desk. I'm a few feet away in the armchair.

'You've accepted you have a problem. This is the place to cry. We'll pick you up. You need that release.'

I've softened to the point of having tears in my eyes but I stop them falling.

I tell Christina that according to his psychologist, my PTSD has deeply affected my youngest son Harry. Patrick has probably internalised his distress. Outwardly, Belle is doing better, but she is intuitive, quick to notice when something is wrong.

Christina doesn't seem surprised, nor does she sugar-coat. She says my levels of arousal – state of alert and response to unexpected noise – will be always higher than people who don't have PTSD. I need to understand how my body works, recognise when I'm agitated, angry or anxious. The idea is to communicate what's happening before I'm unreachable. Mary and the kids need a code word to use when they see me getting wound up, so I can take steps to calm myself. And if I leave the room suddenly, I need to return later, after I'm feeling better, to explain why.

I can't grasp the idea of having PTSD forever, so I push it to one side. But code words make sense. My abrupt disappearances at home worry Mary and confuse the kids. I simply don't know how to articulate what's going on inside my head, my body. I nod at Christina. 'I can do code words,' I say.

PTSD comes with a dizzying array of symptoms. I rank nightmares, flashbacks, anxiety, agitation, depression and noise sensitivity about equal on the impact scale. The worst for me is rage, with emotional numbness just below. My numbness grew as a natural defence mechanism, as Maryam told me, when I covered the Bali bombings. It was in the Mount Elizabeth Hospital in Singapore the following month, not long after Harry's birth, that Mary noticed something was wrong.

Mary had planned to have Harry in Tasmania but after the bombings she didn't want to be too far from Patrick, whose adoption wasn't finished, so we chose Singapore.

Life was never the same in Indonesia after the attacks. Heavily armed police guarded international schools, hotels and shopping centres. We pulled Patrick out of pre-school. Jeremy Wagstaff and his partner Sari Sudarsono stayed at our house to mind him when I flew to Singapore the day before Mary was scheduled for a C-section. As Mary figured Harry would be the only child she'd have, she wanted me there to witness and feel the miracle of birth. But for this to happen, we'd need to set a date.

I'd been spending long hours in the office, covering the hunt for the Bali bombers and their links to al-Qaeda. World events were becoming defining factors in our lives. I was excited about becoming a father again, but something felt off in the hospital: the smell of antiseptic, the equipment, the masks and gowns worn by the doctors and nurses. I missed the chaos of Jakarta, the newsroom hum.

I held Mary's hand as her obstetrician worked behind a small curtain. Harry announced his arrival at 6.01 pm with a roar then fell asleep. He weighed 3.88 kilograms (8.55 pounds). I proudly cradled my beautiful son then placed him in Mary's arms. After a couple of hours, I went back to our hotel, telling Mary I wanted to rest. I didn't return until the next morning.

What sort of father, what sort of husband does that?

Without knowing it, I'd shut down my capacity to feel, to touch, to love, to live.

I love my family, but feel disconnected from them, I tell Christina.

'It's like my heart is frozen. I desperately want to change that.'

'Recognising and acknowledging you are numb is important,' she replies.

Since my first session with Maryam, I've tried to recall who I was before numbness encased me. Who was this man Mary married? Was I like that before? Why did Mary say yes?

Christina wants to talk about my marriage. I go straight to sex, which is pathetic. There has been little intimacy in recent years, I say. I want to make love more with Mary. I also just want to cuddle in bed, but Mary won't.

'I think she worries I'll want sex every time,' I say.

Mary and I had a wonderful sex life in the years after we met. If one of us had been travelling, even if only for a few days, we'd make love almost immediately upon being reunited. It was like we couldn't get back into a routine until we'd been pressed against each other. Waking up next to her was a dream.

But in recent years, Mary had been more tired and distant as she tried to navigate my moods. Of course, she had three children on her hands, was studying full-time, and her elderly parents had bought a house next door to us in Evandale, and they needed her attention.

Again, Christina shows no surprise.

'Men with PTSD need to be physically soothed sometimes

but their partners are always on guard, hypervigilant for any unpredictability, anger, agitation or mood swings towards them or their children,' she says.

'Because of that, women find it difficult to be intimate from any perspective, from hugging to having sex. They can't just flick a switch. You and Mary need to communicate better. This is where most PTSD marriages break down, failure to talk, then alienation. And violence or the threat of violence from men plays a big part too.'

I know this conversation won't go anywhere unless Christina knows everything.

I tell her about the first time I cheated on Mary. We were based in Hanoi and had been together for nearly five years. Mary was reporting TV stories in Vietnam's south. I got drunk with friends including two Australian diplomats. I went to a nightclub called Apocalypse Now after the movie of the same name, drank more, and then got on the back of a motorbike with a sex worker and went to her place. The alcohol removed any moral restraints. I'd visited sex workers before I met Mary, in Indonesia and Australia.

The next morning at home I couldn't remember what happened. I might have had unprotected sex. I didn't carry a condom. I knew I had to tell Mary, but I needed to talk to someone first. My closest friends in Vietnam were the two diplomats, both women my age. They lived around the corner in a quasi-compound. Both agreed I had to tell Mary. One said Mary would understand, the other said she'd leave me.

I got a taxi to the airport and flew to Ho Chi Minh City, where Mary was. It was a Saturday or a Sunday. I called Mary, said I wanted to see her.

In her hotel room, I nervously told Mary what I'd done, what I couldn't remember, how sorry I was.

'Please don't leave me,' I said.

Mary forgave me and blamed herself.

'It's my fault. I haven't been around enough, I'm not meeting your physical needs,' she said.

'No, I'm at fault,' I replied.

I truly believed the blame was mine. But what I took from the conversation, and it's a terrible thing, was that I could satisfy my physical desires if Mary was travelling. I just had to be more careful. I attached no emotion to the thought process, which is beyond fucked given how much I loved and admired my beautiful wife.

Mary was often exhausted when our kids were young, and her depression affected her libido. So I justified occasionally going for massages with extra services at five-star hotels in Jakarta by telling myself I wasn't causing tension at home by pressuring Mary and that I wasn't cheating on her emotionally.

But when I finished my Baghdad bureau chief posting and we moved to Singapore in late 2008, something snapped. I had this sudden and constant urge to be penetrated by a sex toy and have anal sex with Mary. These urges had been building. I could feel it every time I came home for breaks from Baghdad, when Mary and the kids were living in Australia. She hated both but sometimes reluctantly agreed.

The extramarital sex meant nothing, I tell Christina. I never had an affair with another woman. I was never tempted, never flirted all the years I travelled. I'm not trying to absolve myself, just make a distinction. I didn't see my behaviour as shameful.

Christina and I have been talking for 90 minutes. It's dark outside. I'm drained. Christina says she will speak to Mary in a couple of days. 'You can mention anything I've said,' I say.

*

That night I tell Mary I had a good chat with Christina, which reassures her. She knows I've connected with my treating team. I want to talk about intimacy, but before I can, Mary apologises for the 'no ripple effect' comment when we spoke on my first night in Ward 17. She won't say it again. Mary must have sensed it had hurt me, even though we'd agreed to say exactly what was on our minds.

Mary says she has an appointment with a psychologist coming up but feels guilty because the focus must be on me.

'You're the one who's really suffering, not me,' she says.

I've learnt from my treating team that a partner should never play down the impact on them. I say this to Mary without pressing the issue. On one level I knew my trauma had deeply affected Mary and my kids. But my understanding of PTSD and moral injury is still limited. It will take years to fully reflect on and acknowledge the impact of what I've done to my family, especially Mary.

A few days later, Mary texts to say she has sent me an email and could I please read it. Her tone is unusual. I open it with trepidation.

Help Baby,

I feel I'm inflicting more misery on you. To do so, cuts me like a knife. But I know that now is the time to say these things in order to heal . . .

In the years during and after you covered the Bali bombings, Aceh, Israel and Iraq, our sex life changed a lot . . . I didn't really understand what this was about, and I suppose I felt it was something lacking in me. But something told me this wasn't quite normal unless you were into bondage, and I wasn't. I began to avoid sex and at one stage even encouraged you to get satisfaction elsewhere because I didn't feel I was enough. But that was a destructive thing to do . . .

I wonder if the change in sex was part of PTSD? You were self-medicating with the sort of sex that enabled you to escape things. I have to say all this now because if I don't, it will never be said. And now is the time for us to heal and not, in my case, hide behind things that are too hard to say. I know that in bringing these things up I risk hurting you and damaging our relationship, but I think we both need to accept that. If our relationship is going to survive this – and I know we love each other deeply – we need to be really honest with one another. And I know that you have been with me.

I'm sorry for all the pain this email will cause you, babe. It's cold comfort for you but I have cried and cried as I typed.

I close my eyes. Guilt rips through me. I'm causing all our problems. Mary is showing enormous vulnerability. I print off the email, go back to my room and call her. I've wanted to have this conversation for days. It's as if Mary read my mind because she hasn't spoken to Christina yet.

'No one is to blame,' she says.

I breathe deeply.

'I'm glad you are being so honest,' I reply, relieved.

I hear relief in her voice, too. I sense we can work this out.

We have a short, but good conversation. Mary needs to head out. Both of us are speaking separately to Christina later. I make a mental note to talk to Maryam about whether my obsession with the sex Mary hated was connected to PTSD. I also send Mary's email, with her permission, to Maryam and Christina.

Mary wrote her email after reading *Irritable Hearts: A PTSD Love Story,* by American journalist Gabriel Mac, formerly Mac

96

McClelland, that was published in 2015. Mac developed PTSD after reporting on the endemic rape of women following the 2010 earthquake in Haiti that killed 300,000 people. Mac's career as a human rights reporter had taken him to dark corners of the world and exposed him to much personal risk, none more so than in Haiti. Living as a woman at the time, Mac later found that he couldn't process the thought of having sex without violence. During the day, he thought of getting choked and hit while fighting back. 'All I want is to have incredibly violent sex,' Mac told his therapist. For whatever reason, Mac wrote, his body needed this. In his book, Mac recounted the emails he got from traumatised people – rape survivors to veterans – who understood why.

Mac's book also reminded Mary of the 2005 film *Munich*, which we'd watched together years earlier. The movie stars Australian actor Eric Bana, who plays an Israeli Mossad agent called Avner leading a years-long mission to find and kill many of the Palestinian militants who took eleven Israeli athletes and coaches hostage at the 1972 Munich Olympics. All the Israelis were killed. In the final scene, his mission over, Avner is lying in bed with his wife, staring vacantly at the ceiling. Avner's wife reaches out, touches his face, strokes his hair, trying to bring him back to the present. She initiates lovemaking. When the camera shows Avner on top of his wife, he's in a place of shocking violence and trauma. His expression is twisted and tortured. He thrusts into his wife, screaming, sweat flying off his body.

I see Christina at the end of the day after she has spoken with Mary.

'You have to work out this intimacy issue or it might destroy you both,' she says.

In my next session with Maryam – who has read Mary's email – I tell her I think that in Singapore I wanted to feel pain. Because I was numb, maybe I wanted to feel something, anything. This is part of PTSD, Maryam says. My guilt and shame over what happened in Iraq was also a factor, she believes. I wanted to be punished.

'But as for Mary encouraging you to find sex elsewhere, that's not consent, that's coercion,' Maryam says with uncharacteristic firmness. 'Mary had no choice. And you cannot expect a woman to be aroused if her partner has been agitated all day and her kids have been on edge.'

I hadn't seen it that way until then. Maryam was right. I had coerced Mary.

Being told by someone I respected deeply that I'd coerced Mary was difficult to hear. I tried not to think about this too much because to me coercion implied undue pressure or force. I couldn't face the reality of what I'd done. This probably explains why I wrote nothing about it in my journal aside from the bare-bones of what Maryam said.

The *DSM-5*, published in 2013, added a new symptom of PTSD: reckless or self-destructive behaviour. This could include risky sexual activity. In his book *War and the Soul: Healing our Nation's Veterans from Post-Traumatic Stress Disorder,* American clinical psychotherapist Edward Tick writes that developing an abnormal sex drive is one example of how war can transform someone's relationship to love and passion. He quotes a Vietnam veteran, a medic called Ray, who said: 'I touched more dead bodies in one year than live ones in my entire lifetime.' The desperation of Ray's sexuality when he returned from Vietnam frightened his wife and made her feel dirty. Ray was so deeply imprinted with death that he needed sex to feel the touch of life again. Tick describes another veteran who came back from Vietnam with a hunger for the 'restoration of life that only the intensity of erotic arousal' could fulfill. He insisted on sex at least three times a day, 'any way, anywhere, any time'. He found other women and lived a double life. Finally, his wife felt shamed and used. The ex-marine divorced her to continue his exploits. Lust awakened by war for bloodletting easily transfers to sexuality back home, writes Tick. The wife feels debased. The man justified, as if he is acting of necessity.

In late December 2012, a few weeks before we left Singapore for Tasmania, Mary arranged to meet me at a Starbucks outlet while I was working. Over coffee, she said she'd stay with me as long as I bought her a birthday present every year, just something small. And no more sex workers. Mary felt neglected when I hadn't bought her a gift, and I never forgot once we got to Tasmania.

I knew my marriage was on the line over the sex workers and I promised Mary I'd stop. I meant it. The previous month we'd seen this beautiful one-storey brick homestead in Evandale for sale on the internet. Mary flew down from Singapore the next day to inspect the house. We bought it hours later. I celebrated that afternoon by going to a brothel. During sex, the condom burst. What should have been a memorable day was forever tarnished because I had to tell Mary when she got back to Singapore. I went on an expensive 28-day course of drugs (post-exposure prophylaxis, or PEP) to reduce the possibility of HIV transmission.

But I couldn't shake the reckless behaviour described in the *DSM-5*, even if it was nothing like on the scale of Singapore. Mary's ultimatum in Starbucks was a pivotal moment in the

28 years we have been together. Yet I still crossed her line. When I look back, I was emotionally numb to those around me, especially Mary. My heart was frozen, as I said to Christina. But the fucking recklessness of my actions, the risks I took, beggar belief. I could have destroyed our family.

—

About halfway through my admission, I agree with Maryam that I should fly home for a long weekend. Maryam sees my trip as a test run before I'm discharged at the end of week five. I want to stay longer. No, this can't be a refuge, she replies.

Mary wants to see me but is nervous. I am too but my trauma knowledge is growing and I have strategies to deal with stress at home. Mary is getting great support from Jeremy, his wife Sari and a British friend, Tessa Piper, who lives in Jakarta. Jeremy set up a WhatsApp group chat that excluded me so Mary could talk openly. Their first exchange on 29 August comes a couple of days before I go home.

Mary: *I don't know what's wrong with me today. I had a bad parenting day yesterday and feel so guilty and awful. I'm sitting behind my computer crying . . . Feeling sorry for myself when Dean is being so brave.*

Tessa: *You are dealing with so much. It's amazing you are keeping everything together.*

Jeremy: *I second that . . . You're looking after three kids, a house, parents, chooks, dog, cats, have I left anyone out?*

Sari: *Sorry to hear that, Sis . . . Here is some love for you from me, your spiritual companion.* 😄😌💚🖤💚❤️❤️❤️😳😳😳

Mary: *Thanks Sari. I suppose I'll laugh later about Patrick*

100

storming out of mum and dad's place because I took his birthday cake over to have as a family. He's too big to smack.

Jeremy: *Oh dear, that doesn't sound like a kodak moment . . .*

Mary: *Ok, I'm laughing now! Thank you! I can get through the day. Dean's psychiatrist told him that when he comes home it will be the first test of how he's doing. I'm very worried because I know there'll be many triggers. I worry he'll come home and we'll find it's the same situation and it'll be very demoralising for us both.*

Jeremy: *I think he knows he's still in the first stage of the process (can't remember the others). So, I don't think his expectations will be high, or that he thinks there's some magical moment when he's 'fixed'. Just try to make it as normal as possible, let him enjoy some decent food and a few drinks (is he allowed them?). He's the one who recognises he needs longer in there so I think he knows that any sign of improvement, however small, will be good, but not to expect too much . . .*

Sari: *Jeremy is right. His PTSD happened over many years. His recovery WILL also take time.*

Mary: *Excellent advice! I can't expect there aren't going to be triggers and tense moments.*

Tessa: *I would add that the toughest thing for you, Mary, (among many) will be trying not to be too anxious about everything . . . This isn't all on you to fix.*

Mary: *Yes you're right. Our lives are never going to be the same again.*

Jeremy: *And I think Dean is close to a revelation where he will kick into a whole new gear. It will take a while – could be a year – but he'll be v fulfilled, maybe more than he has been in years.*

Mary: *I just feel so tired. I've been living on adrenalin and know all my senses will kick into hyper-vigilance again waiting to stop that door slamming, or the dog barking at shadows or to catch falling plates or take back anything the children and I say that hasn't come out right. My gut clenches at the thought. But I'm not the one who had to live under constant mortar fire and shoulder the horror of losing 3 staff in Baghdad, or wade through the bodies of women and children in Aceh. So, I go back to my point at the beginning. Anything I say is just so self-indulgent. How do families get through this? I suppose they just learn to live with it and carve out a new identity.*

Jeremy: *I think however much it doesn't feel like it, there's progress. It's slow but it's there.*

Tessa: *And try to stop feeling that what you and the children are going through is nothing compared to the horrors Dean experienced. It's of course very different but what you are dealing with is huge emotionally. And you are feeling the additional burden of trying to keep everything and everyone going.*

—

I buy good headphones at the airport and find a quiet corner to listen to music while waiting for my flight. Breathing in and out through my nose keeps my anxiety under control. I'm desperate for the weekend to go smoothly. I've sent Mary a note with my 'objectives', a sign the methodical news agency journalist is back. They include:

- Work out code words in case my anxiety escalates.
- Mentally prepare myself for the dog barking. Calm her myself or leave the room and do breathing exercises.
- Explain to the kids my routine in Ward 17.
- Make Sunday a lovely birthday for Mary.
- Walk around the garden with Mary each evening.
- Talk about intimacy, but the weekend is not about sex (presumptuous, I know), it's about being close.

Sheep and cows are grazing on farmland as Evandale comes into view, patches of water on the surface from recent rain. Mary and I embrace before getting into the car at the airport. I breathe in the air, the lack of people and buildings. Within minutes we're home. Mary's tulips and daffodils are in bloom. Blossoms on the trees. Spring!

Belle jumps up and down when she sees me. Patrick and Harry are more restrained. When I wake the following morning, I tell Mary I'm anxious. She knows; I look terrible. But now she doesn't have to guess. I explain to Harry I had to face my fears outside the glass door at Ward 17. I'm getting good treatment. Patrick has the flu, so he stays in his room, though I cook his meals. Belle and I roast a leg of lamb for lunch for Mary's birthday.

Mary and I hold each other in bed at night and in the morning. I tell her how much I love moving my hand from her side to her hip and thigh and back. She quips about her weight and age.

'I love feeling you because it's *you*,' I say.

I need to convince Mary that being with her is what matters. What neither of us realises yet is that her body will remember what I've done.

On my first night home, I take two Valium tablets to sleep. The second and third nights, nothing. Is it the closeness in bed with Mary? Or the little voice in my head saying: don't worry, you'll soon be back in Ward 17.

I tell Mary in detail for the first time what happened in the Singapore brothels, how I wanted to get tied up and flogged but couldn't find anyone to do it. Mary says she wouldn't get close to me in bed because she was afraid of the sex I'd want. She drank a bottle of wine every night and slept in the spare room. I don't remember this. The anal sex was painful, she adds, it hurt for days.

Mary agrees with Maryam's assessment that I wanted to be punished and that I had coerced her. She felt so confused over who I'd become that she didn't see it as coercion at the time. She loved me and didn't want our marriage to end because she knew I was lost and would find my way back if she just hung on.

Some people might ask why Mary didn't talk to me about this. She feared an eruption. Our kids were young and had their own challenges.

Mary then reminds me about the condom-bursting incident and her ultimatum in Starbucks. I tell Mary how sorry I am for hurting her so much. I ask if she'd like to sell the house to help remove the stain over our relationship. She says no. Again, I hope we can resolve things by talking. I don't have the courage to tell her I haven't kept my promise.

It will be years before I truly open my heart to the searing pain my infidelity inflicted on Mary. Integrate her feelings into my deeply thought-through ideas on trauma and healing. Our relationship deserved the same attention I devoted to grappling with the deaths of my Iraqi staff.

I convinced myself that I'd never cheated on Mary emotionally, that the sex meant nothing. Shame will come crashing in when I fully realise I'm not the only one in our house who has been deeply betrayed. But this will also be liberating because it allows Mary and me to rebuild. We talk so much about what happened and why. We will leave no stone unturned.

Barely a day goes by now where I don't think about my remarkable partner, how lucky I am, and try to express this in some way. Intimacy is so much more than sex. Emotional numbness and male privilege have made way for the man I am proud to be.

Some level of shame will always be with me, and I'm good with that. It's a healthy dose.

9

The moral dimension of trauma

Dr Maryam listened to me talk about Namir and Saeed in our first session. At the end of our second meeting, she asked me to write down what I thought I should have done for them. That afternoon I re-read the email exchanges I'd had with my old Baghdad colleagues in recent weeks. I looked at my notes from phone conversations, my chats with Mary, my journal entries.

I'd repeatedly asked myself if I did enough to investigate Namir and Saeed's deaths. I'd evaluated what all sides said – legal experts, journalists, former Apache pilots, soldiers from the 2nd Battalion, 16th Infantry Regiment – both in published stories and on social media. I'd gone over and over the transcript of the pilot banter. I must surely have read that permission was given to Crazy Horse 1–8 to open fire before Namir peered around the corner, but it hasn't registered. All I see is an image of Namir, frozen in time, from that military briefing in Baghdad nine years earlier.

*

A month ago, on the eve of the ninth anniversary of Namir and Saeed's deaths, my body itched all over as I tried to sleep. I got up and sat by the wood-fired heater in the living room. Mary came out and put her arm around me.

'What's going through your mind?' she asked.

'I think I'm closer to understanding why I feel such guilt and shame,' I replied. 'Irrespective of how suspicious Namir looked, did that Apache have the right to open fire? The way I reacted at the briefing would say yes.'

'What do you mean?' said Mary.

'The way I put my head in my hands. I was blaming Namir. Is this wrong? It feels wrong now. I feel guilty for even thinking Namir's actions caused that tragic loss of life,' I said.

'The other thing is the tape. I should have fought harder to get it. I should have stood up at press conferences in Baghdad and demanded a copy, saying journalist safety was at stake. And why didn't I do anything about Reuters' pathetic response to its release? Why didn't I write the full story of what happened? Why did I hide?'

I didn't feel any emotion that night, though. I had no clue what to do with the discovery. I also had no recollection of the global outcry over the release of Collateral Murder. Emptiness continued to consume me the next morning, the anniversary, but to Mary's surprise my mood improved. I looked forward to paying my respects to Namir, Saeed and translator Lu'oy al-Joubouri.

That evening I lit scented candles Mary had bought for them. I spread the red, white and black Iraqi flag on the kitchen table. It was the first time I'd unfolded it since I left Baghdad. My staff had written heartfelt messages on the flag. Yasser Faisal said: 'I wish you happiness and great health always to your family.' Yasser was a cameraman for Reuters from 2003 to 2009. He was killed in Syria on 4 December 2013, while on assignment for a Spanish media company. Muhanad Mohammed wrote: 'I wish to our Great God to keep you from harm because you are a good man.' Muhanad was a driver then a reporter for eight years. He was killed in a suicide bombing in Baghdad on 19 December 2013. I was deeply fond of both men.

If only Yasser and Muhanad knew the real Dean, the man who failed to protect their colleagues, failed to speak up when he should have.

I wrote to a former Iraqi colleague, Waleed Ibrahim, the day after the anniversary. Waleed had translated for me when the young cameraman burst through the door with news that Namir and Saeed had been killed. Waleed and I used to watch English Premier League games together on Saturday afternoons if it wasn't busy. It was the first time I'd been in touch with Waleed in six years, since Julian Assange published Collateral Murder and Waleed told me the Iraqi staff were outraged, believing I'd seen the whole tape and done nothing. That email exchange nearly broke my heart. Waleed is now Iraq bureau chief for Al Jazeera.

'One of the things that troubles me most is guilt,' I said to Waleed. 'Guilt that I didn't do enough to prevent Namir and Saeed from being killed. Guilt that I believed Namir was acting suspiciously when he pointed his camera around that corner. Guilt that I didn't pursue our case against the US military hard enough. Guilt that I didn't stand up and be counted when WikiLeaks released the video in 2010 that showed Namir and Saeed's horrible, horrible deaths. Guilt that when I left Baghdad I abandoned all my wonderful friends . . . I need to hear from people like you, Waleed, how you really felt. I need people to be honest with me.'

None of it was your fault, Waleed said. It was Namir and Saeed's fate, their destiny, in accordance with Islamic beliefs.

I pressed Waleed, asking what the Iraqi staff expected me to do.

'I need to know how I should have responded so I can reach some sort of acceptance of my actions, then try to move on.'

Waleed replied: 'None of the Iraqi staff ever thought that you let them down over Namir and Saeed. It wasn't your mistake. It was their fate to come under the fire of a savage and barbarian American pilot. I beg you, don't think in this way and burden yourself.'

Going over all this material helps me gather my thoughts. I write Maryam a 900-word summary of the many things I failed to do, including that I never asked US military contacts about the rules of engagement for Iraq.

Sitting in our usual patient–therapist room, Maryam takes my note and reads it.

'I cheated my staff into thinking I was something I wasn't. I abandoned them when I left Baghdad and again when the WikiLeaks video was released,' I say.

I'm expecting a robust debate, but Maryam doesn't ask any questions. Instead, she wants me to later write down the good things I've done for my staff in various postings over the years. I'm a bit surprised. Helping a Vietnamese news assistant get a Fulbright scholarship to the United States won't make up for two dead men, I think to myself.

Maryam senses I'm sceptical about the new exercise.

'It's not about changing your feelings. It's about getting you to see the other side. I want you to have some perspective.'

Maryam then blows my mind by saying she has watched

Collateral Murder. I hadn't even thought of asking her to do so. Before I can respond, Maryam says I'm not well enough to view it and probably won't be at any point during my admission.

'What do you mean? The longer I leave it the harder it gets.'

Maryam says my arousal levels are too high to watch Collateral Murder. I need to stabilise first, understand my triggers. She also thinks I want to punish myself by watching the tape.

'You need to learn to live with what happened,' Maryam says.

I can see Maryam won't budge on the tape (again), so I tell her about my plan to be in Baghdad for the tenth anniversary of Namir and Saeed's deaths next year. I'll go to London first to see Namir's older brother Nabeel. Saeed's family are in Baghdad. Namir's parents live in Mosul, which is controlled by Islamic State, one of the many deadly legacies of the US occupation. I'll work out how to deal with that logistical issue later.

'I used to think five years ahead, my brain was so organised. My only thought now is being in Baghdad. Otherwise, there is nothing. I need to stand with the families and honour them,' I say.

'Will Reuters let you go?' asks Maryam.

'They can't stop me,' I reply.

Maryam says I need to learn how to live with what she calls a scar.

Several days later, I ask how I can possibly move on. 'You're processing, it will take time,' she says. 'Don't be impatient, your mind is moving too fast.'

PTSD has broad recognition across society even if its full reach and impact is poorly understood. While the term is only 43 years old, it's had many names since armies fought in Ancient Greece. Trauma is the Greek word for wound, a physical one, although these days the context is often emotional or psychological. What we know of as PTSD was called soldier's or irritable heart in the American Civil War. Shell shock described men who broke down under fire in the trenches of World War One.

Moral injury is far more obscure but also has its genesis on the battlefields of Ancient Greece. American psychiatrist Jonathan Shay coined the term in the mid-1990s after years of treating Vietnam War veterans with severe PTSD. It's not that Shay didn't think his patients had PTSD. But what he witnessed was something beyond the well-known combat scenarios of life-threat and fear: it was an indignant rage in men betrayed by their commanders in Vietnam *and* when they got home. He believed veterans could usually recover from the horror, fear and grief of war if their notion of 'what's right' hadn't been violated.

Shay gave the example of soldiers who killed Vietnamese fish-ermen and children because of bad intelligence but who were given medals because they got 'body count'. American soldiers experienced such betrayal repeatedly in Vietnam, their experi-ences erased and denied. Back home they were not honoured, were treated with indifference or derision.

As Shay put it, he saw the absence of dignity in the indignant rage of his patients. He settled on the definition of moral injury as the betrayal of what's right by someone who holds legitimate authority (for example, a military superior) in a high-stakes situa-tion. Shay drew parallels between his veterans and warriors from Ancient Greece, in particular Homer's epic poems the *Iliad* and the *Odyssey*.

Moral injury remained a fringe concept until clinicians and researchers led by Brett Litz, a professor in the departments of psychiatry and psychology at Boston University, published an academic paper in 2009 that defined a second form of the condition among US veterans: 'Perpetrating, failing to prevent, bearing witness to, or learning about acts that transgress deeply held moral beliefs and expectations. This may entail participating in or witnessing inhumane or cruel actions, failing to prevent the immoral acts of others, as well as engaging in subtle acts or experiencing reactions that, upon reflection, transgress a moral code.'

Soldiers and veterans could suffer long-term wounds that were not well captured by the PTSD formulation, the authors wrote in the 2009 paper. The clinical science community had given little heed to moral wounds, they added, possibly because of the focus on the impact of life-threat trauma.

The commander, the powerholder, was the violator in Shay's definition of moral injury. It was the ordinary soldier for Litz and his colleagues.

Litz will tell me at the end of the year that journalists can suffer moral injury too.

I'm trying to understand where PTSD and moral injury intersect and differ. There appears to be some agreement among experts that they can co-exist and also that it's possible to have one and not the other. PTSD is classified as a mental illness under the *DSM-5* but moral injury is not, partly because the research base is tiny and has been confined mainly to US veterans. Moral injury does, however, have many of the same symptoms as PTSD, and in some ways is more difficult to heal from.

—

It's a Friday afternoon and Ward 17 is quiet with many patients on weekend leave. I'm in the third week of my admission. I love my morning walks to the stream, where I stop and watch the ducks. I say hi to other walkers, notice the blossoms coming out on the trees. I've shared everything with my treating team, bonded with the veterans, coppers and other patients. Mary and I talk each day about what I'm learning.

I've been thinking about people I worked with over the years in Baghdad, Jerusalem, Gaza, Jakarta, Hanoi and other places. I miss the closeness, the camaraderie. I think it's because the vets and coppers have made me feel so welcome. Summer evenings in Baghdad, eating Masgouf fish and drinking Coronas in the Reuters compound while the war was going on. The Irish security guards would take me to the Green Zone and we'd fill the boot of the bureau's armour-plated BMW with alcohol. I'd expense it as 'beverages'. Last week when thinking about how much these people meant to me I even felt teary, which is not me! Is this loss? Am I mourning something? When colleagues at the BBC were unhurt after a rocket hit their house in May 2008 in Baghdad, the Associated Press (AP) threw a party in their neighbouring compound the following night. It was a celebration of life. We competed fiercely on the story, but collective safety came first. It was the only time I got drunk in Baghdad. Another fond memory: a Saturday afternoon, after nearly a week of reporting an earthquake on Indonesia's Nias Island in March 2004 that killed 1000 people, the AP's Chris Brummitt and I decided we'd had enough. Chris had also covered the Boxing Day tsunami three months earlier. We found a kiosk selling beer, sat on a little wharf that hadn't been damaged in the quake and drank all afternoon. We didn't bother to tell our editors.

I get up from my green hospital armchair, go to my desk and start typing.

Does this forensic review of my actions matter now? Is it important? What will I achieve? I know deep down that the Apache pilot seemed genuine when he saw Namir peer around the corner. He believed Namir was about to fire, even though you can ask, 'Does a long-lens camera really look like an RPG?' But Namir did look suspicious. Does that justify unleashing such firepower? This is one reason why I need to watch the WikiLeaks video.

Could I have lobbied harder for the tape? Yes, I could have stood up at press conferences. I don't think I did because it wasn't my style and I believed we'd get the tape. I was wrong.

I was gutless. I froze. I could have convinced Reuters we needed a much stronger response. Saeed was alive, for fuck's sake, when the Apache opened fire again. Maybe he could have been saved.

I just wanted someone else to deal with it. I should have written a story that set the record straight. This was my greatest failing. What's important now? Getting on with life? Reconnecting with my family? Paying respects to Namir and Saeed? Atoning?

And I just had a crazy thought. What about the Apache crew? Are they remorseful? Got PTSD? I'd feel compassion for them if they do.

I sit back in my chair and look out the window at the gum trees. My screen is all consciousness and typos. Where did that come from?

Fuck it. It's time to tell the truth. I was cowardly when Assange released the video. I was shocked but wanted someone else to deal with it. I dishonoured myself. That's what I must live with, atone for. *This* is my moral injury.

I shut my laptop, put my earphones in and walk to Ivanhoe to buy fish and chips for dinner. My thoughts need to settle.

I type the notes up properly over the weekend and email them to Maryam. Not sure where I'm going with this, be good to discuss, I say.

Maryam is pleased when I see her on Monday, says I'm making progress, being less hard on myself. She says it makes sense that my thoughts crystallised as I wrote. I think I'm starting to come to some sort of acceptance, I say. Maryam, perceptive as ever, asks if what I'm feeling is more here (she points to her head) than here (at her heart). I nod.

A week later I tell her that Namir and Saeed no longer dominate my mind. I've stopped reading my Baghdad emails, even stopped obsessing about watching Collateral Murder. Maryam suggests all the talking and thinking is helping me process. I'm structuring these thoughts and learning to cope with them better.

In her notes, Maryam writes that she suspects I feel guilty for not thinking about Namir and Saeed as much.

I tell her I've been reading about therapy for soldiers and veterans with moral injury called Adaptive Disclosure that Litz and his colleagues have developed. They published a book earlier in the year: *Adaptive Disclosure: A New Treatment for Military Trauma, Loss and Moral Injury*. I've ordered a copy. The distress their patients suffer reflects a fair appraisal of culpability and responsibility from the warzone, they argue. Self-condemnation and guilt are natural consequences of the emotional agony of an intact moral compass. Rather than help veterans extinguish fear or challenge their beliefs about what happened – core elements to treating PTSD – Adaptive Disclosure takes a different approach. It focuses on acceptance, seeking forgiveness, self-compassion and finding meaning from trauma as the pathway to moral repair. One route might be dialogue with a forgiving moral authority. Vets might seek to make amends, in real terms, or symbolically. They are also encouraged to write letters, either apologising to the person they believe they wronged or confiding in a trusted friend or spiritual leader. They don't have to send the letters.

Just writing helps them connect with their compassionate side, a part they might have lost.

'I want to write a letter to Namir and Saeed,' I tell Maryam.

Maryam gets animated even before I can finish the sentence.

'It's a great idea,' she says, leaning forward in her chair, smiling. 'I think you feel there is much you need to say, words inside your mind and heart that you haven't said. This will be a way of getting the emotions out.'

Little do I know how hard it will be to write that letter or how important it will be to making peace with myself.

10

Soldier D

About 3 am on Friday 9 September, loud screaming jolts me awake. At breakfast, copper Matt Ross says he heard it too. Matt's room is next to mine. He reckons it was Soldier D, a big veteran aged about 40 who sleeps in a room around the corner. Soldier D is one of the most popular patients in Ward 17. He makes us laugh at mealtimes or in the evening when we relax on the couches. He treats the kitchen staff like family.

A little while later, Soldier D sits down with toast and a cup of tea. The fit six-foot three-inch young warrior who moonlighted as a bouncer in Sydney's roughest nightspots in the late 1990s disappeared long ago. The groggy man sitting opposite me probably weighs 120 kilograms. Military tattoos cover his body. Bags drop from his eyes.

'Sorry about that. Nightmares. Hope I didn't wake anyone,' Soldier D says, his usual sunniness gone.

A few hours later I'm reading in my room when the song 'Dirty Deeds Done Dirt Cheap' by AC/DC crashes through my end of Ward 17. That's ballsy, I think. The unit manager runs a tight ship. Minutes later, alarms sound. A voice over the hospital PA says:

'Code Blue, Ward 17.'

I open my door. Through the small internal garden courtyard, I see staff racing down the opposite corridor. Headed for Soldier D's room, I figure.

It's nearly lunchtime. Most patients have left for weekend leave. I sit with Matt and several others on the couches around the coffee table. OT Michelle comes over to check on us. Matt and I say we're fine.

Matt is a quirky copper, funny, has a long beard. I haven't seen him show a single symptom of PTSD. A veteran of highway patrol, Matt has told me it's not fatal accidents that get him, but screaming children trapped in cars. Because he doesn't have children, he tells the coppers on shift with him that do have kids to direct traffic.

Matt and I are not fine, but we're both wearing our professional masks, copper and journo. A few other patients are shaking badly. Michelle arranges for nurses to give them Valium. I follow Michelle as she walks away.

Is Soldier D alive? I ask quietly.

Yes, she replies.

Half an hour later, emergency staff wheel Soldier D out of Ward 17 on his bed. We can't see Soldier D from where we sit. We don't know what's happened.

———

Soldier D grew up in Queenstown on Tasmania's sparsely populated west coast. The town is famous for a landscape denuded

117

by more than a century of mining and smelting. Mining began around Queenstown in 1883. When gold was exhausted in 1891, attention turned to a huge copper deposit. The Mount Lyell mine operated continuously until 2014, when production stopped after the deaths of three miners in two accidents. The town is a long drive from Launceston or Hobart. The last hour or so on either journey winds through sections of thick rainforest. There is a strange beauty to Queenstown and its old frontier buildings. Mist often covers the lunar-like hills because of heavy west coast rainfall. But it can be a tough, isolated place to live.

Soldier D loved exploring the west coast wilderness growing up. He fished, hunted and played Australian rules football. At breakfast one day early in our admissions, we discovered we'd both slept in the same old miner's hut next to Fraser Creek in the Tarkine rainforest. Soldier D had been there nineteen times, as a scout and on school trips.

As much as Soldier D loved the west coast of Tasmania, he didn't want the life of his father, who worked in the mine, so he joined the army at seventeen. His first overseas deployment was to East Timor in 2000 as part of the international peace-keeping force sent to restore order after Indonesian-backed militias destroyed the territory following its independence vote. Most militias fled to neighbouring West Timor when peacekeepers began to arrive.

Soldier D was stationed in Maliana, near the border with West Timor. Militias mortared the base occasionally. One day Soldier D was lowered into a well to retrieve what he thought would be the body of a woman. Halfway up, a limb came loose, causing him to drop the body. When Soldier D went back down, he saw a small hand poking through the water. There were five or six children there too.

A born storyteller with an extraordinary memory, Soldier D is open about his battle with PTSD. He's done interviews with the local radio station in Queenstown. But he says getting old scares him – the thought of still having PTSD and being pushed in a wheelchair at Anzac Day parades. He talks about a Vietnam vet he met in a psych ward in Adelaide four months earlier who'd been diagnosed with PTSD in 1981. 'It frightened the shit out of me. I'd rather die young and strong,' he says.

About six hours after Soldier D was wheeled out of Ward 17, I'm sitting on a couch in the common room, reading a book. It's early evening. Suddenly, Soldier D strides through the glass door, into the common room. Relief surges through me. I jump up and go over and put my arm across his massive shoulders. 'Great to see you, mate,' I say, trying not to stare at the red welt around his neck. A few other patients hear us and come out.

With one of Soldier D's friends who has come to support him, we sit around chatting. While there is serious talk, we also laugh and joke. It's a celebration that Soldier D is still with us.

The doctor running intensive care wanted to keep Soldier D there, but his psychiatrist insisted he return to Ward 17. Familiar faces and surroundings.

Soldier D tells us: 'My psych wanted me to make him a promise. I said I don't make promises. So, he asked if I'd work hard with him for the next forty-eight hours. I said I can do that.'

Only the day before at the weekly community meeting, Soldier D complained about not getting his two cups of veggies at mealtimes. He's trying to lose weight.

Nurses shadow Soldier D's every move for the next 72 hours. He isn't allowed to leave the ward. He jokes about going to bed with one nurse on duty and another there when he wakes.

'Two women in one night! And I don't remember,' he says. It's wonderful to hear his voice echoing from the kitchen area.

Journal entry. Ward 17, Melbourne. Sept 9, 2016: Very intense day. Very emotional. But [Soldier D] is alive. People look out for each other in this place. Doesn't matter who you are.

11

Discharge

With my discharge getting closer, Maryam asks me to draw up personal and work goals with a *realistic* timeframe; her emphasis, not mine. She also wants me to write down what I've achieved in Ward 17. I reflect for the first time on my admission, wondering how many one-hour sessions on the outside equal a month here. When I ask Maryam for her approximation, she looks at me quizzically, then says you can't compare.

I've spent every waking moment in Ward 17 getting to grips with my trauma. I think I'm starting to come to some sort of acceptance over Namir and Saeed and Collateral Murder. I can see the potential for finding meaning in life. I'm learning techniques to control my anxiety and stress. I've not yearned for rum and coke since day four or five. And I've forged bonds with other patients. But the most important breakthrough has been my communication with Mary, knowing I can reconnect with my family. Mary is my anchor.

'I'm feeling a little optimistic for the first time in a long time,'

I say to Maryam about a week before I leave. 'It's not just about getting through the day, it's about what comes next.'

'It scares you, doesn't it?' she says.

'It awakens the sceptic in me.'

How could I go from being suicidal six weeks ago? I ask. I think I'm feeling fraudulent again. Was I that sick to begin with? How come I've made progress when many of my mates in here, some after multiple admissions, seem to be treading water?

Maryam calls me psychologically minded. I've sought self-reflection and personal insight. She says recovery can depend on eagerness to engage with treatment, family support and financial stability.

'I've given you homework and you've done it. Maybe you've over-read a little, but you've put a lot of effort into your recovery. For people like me it's rewarding. It also makes me work harder because you ask so many questions. I think Frankl's book has really helped. You see potential for a lot of meaning in your life.'

But you still have much to process, Maryam cautions.

Despite the emerging optimism, I'm tight across my chest for a couple of days. I try walking, meditating and Valium, but nothing helps. Is this progress real? My treating team sense I'm agitated and advise me to focus on self-regulation, building more insight into the connections between my triggers and elevated moods.

Social worker Christina Sim tells me I've chosen not to be a victim of PTSD. Talk to your kids, tell them you're sorry about what's happened but explain you're feeling better, she adds. This will allow them to express how they've felt. Mary and I have decided not to mention my suicidal ideation to them for now. I tell Christina that visiting sex workers while married to Mary now feels wrong. It's the first time I've felt this way.

On my last full day, Maryam chats with Mary on speaker phone. Coincidentally, Maryam is the Persian and Arabic name for Mary. It's a warm exchange. Maryam summarises my treatment and medication. I've made significant progress, she tells Mary – less anxiety and hypervigilance and fewer nightmares. She says I need to ease back into work. Mary thanks Maryam for the regular phone calls from Christina and the nurses, saying this allowed her to share critical confidential observations. Her only question is, what if I go downhill and refuse to listen to her? I say I'll write a letter giving Mary authority to speak to my GP and a new psychologist in Launceston that Ward 17 has arranged for me to see in early October.

'I think I can manage this. I feel confident,' I say.

I give Maryam a note on my goals and email them to Mary.

- *Have realistic expectations of the initial days/weeks at home. Monitor stress and communicate this with my family. Use code words. Don't get manic. Be self-aware, recognise if I'm getting anxious, angry or agitated. Use calming strategies.*
- *Don't get carried away with other projects.*
- *Continue to improve communication and intimacy with Mary.*
- *Connect with my boys. It will be easy with Belle because she spends far more time with her parents and can sense when something is not right.*
- *Exercise/meditate and do breathing exercises daily.*
- *Lose weight.*
- *Walk around the garden every evening with Mary.*
- *Don't buy rum.*
- *Get back to work part-time after school holidays, in about three to four weeks.*

Sitting alone with Maryam, she says I've gotten through the crisis stage, the first phase of my recovery. She encourages me to work hard with the psychologist in Launceston on my core traumatic memories.

I drift back to Baghdad, early 2004. It's winter, colder than people probably think. One of the Iraqi drivers, I can't remember who, is taking me to cover some bullshit event at a US military base I've never heard of. Traffic thins as we get closer to blast walls, then there are no cars. Something is wrong. No checkpoints, no angled concrete barriers that slow a vehicle down. 'Stop!' I shout. Through the windshield, I see a US soldier behind sandbags hunched over a machine gun pointed at our windscreen. We've come to the exit, not the entrance. 'Don't move,' I tell the driver. If we suddenly reverse, the soldier might open fire, thinking we're suicide bombers with second thoughts.

I slowly open the door and hold up my blue PRESS flak jacket, then get out. I yell 'media' and 'journalist'. The soldier says nothing. I'm not a gun expert, but I think he's looking at me through the scope of a SAW, an M249 squad automatic weapon. The barrel is mounted on a tripod. His weapon can fire 200 rounds a minute.

I walk towards him slowly over gravel, left hand raised, the other holding the flak jacket so he can see the PRESS sign in fluorescent white.

'Hey mate! I'm a journalist!'

He's about twenty metres away. For once I'm glad I don't look Arab.

'Fuck, man, I nearly lit you up!' he shouts.

'A lot of stuff is coming back to you, isn't it?' says Maryam.

Yep.

*

I'm not afraid of going home, but I'll miss my mates in Ward 17. Rather than shun me, the broken veterans, coppers and paramedics treated me like a brother. One by one, they wrote their phone numbers and email addresses in my journal.

I scratch a message in the old coffee table: 'No matter your profession or what caused your trauma, we all have PTSD. No one in Ward 17 is alone. Dean, the journo. Sept 2016.'

———

Mary and I sip red wine as we smell her tulips, daffodils and daphnes on my first evening home. Birdsong fills the air, water rushes along the South Esk River. I tell Patrick, Belle and Harry I feel a lot better. I describe the vets and coppers in Ward 17. The brave journey they are on.

The next day, a Saturday, I feel tired and sleep in the afternoon. That doesn't worry Mary nor myself since I've just got home. We walk around the garden again with wine, sit on one of our wooden bench seats as the sun sets. Anxiety grips my chest that night. I don't know why.

I'm anxious when I wake. Breathing exercises don't help, so I take Valium. I do a guided body scan on our bed but fall asleep before it finishes. On Mary's advice, I move my desk and computer from my small study into our guest room, which looks out on the back garden and the river. I have personal affairs to sort out after five weeks away. Mary suggests I deal with one administrative task a day.

It's different to when I came home a couple of weeks ago. Then I did nothing except spend time with the family and cook. The strain is showing.

While I'm talking with the kids, I'm not tuning into their lives.

I'm still numb, emotionally disconnected. Harry's school issues have come to a head. Harry is bright but has struggled with the academic rigour of the local grammar school and suffered bouts of anxiety, missing about a third of school this year – all since I went on sick leave. Mary believes moving him to a smaller public school with less pressure is best. Harry's psychologist agrees. Harry sees sense in the idea but at thirteen is anxious about change, even though he has mates from his local cricket team and Evandale at the state school. I'm stressed and don't want to get involved. I tell Mary she has my support.

Mainstream school had been horrible for Belle. She struggled to concentrate and complete assignments with due dates at the grammar school. Apart from one kind teacher, we always felt Belle was seen as a problem child in their high-achieving academic and sporting environment. She was shy, going through a period of self-neglect, and found comfort and safety only at home and with animals. When Mary moved Belle to a school for kids with learning difficulties at fourteen, she thrived.

Patrick has just turned sixteen and is in grade 10. Mary and I don't know it yet, but not only is he worried about me, he's lost interest in art, his passion in life. He feels hemmed in at the grammar school, unhappy, and wants to drop the subject. In Singapore, Mary and I knew his art teacher because our kids did swimming training with him on Saturday mornings. One day when Patrick was close to finishing grade 5, the teacher said Patrick had the talent to be an artist. We had no idea. What we did know was Patrick had unusual powers of concentration and a quirky sense of humour.

Patrick will move to a public school for grade 11 where an amazing young female teacher reignites his love of art and introduces him to oil painting.

As if Mary doesn't have enough to deal with, I resume running in my sleep the night I tell her to shoulder Harry's school issues. A couple of nights later I wake with a vice across my chest. My heart races. Breathing exercises and Valium help. Mary gets up at 6 am. I stay in bed a bit longer and dream I'm in Taipei reporting news of a Chinese rocket attack on the city. The ground shakes, people flee. Some buildings topple or are engulfed in fireballs. I stumble out of bed at 7.30 am. Mary says I look awful. I do a body scan and sleep for an hour. *I'm not going to let PTSD spoil my day.*

By midday I feel better. The birdsong soothes me. Not a day has gone by since getting home that I haven't marvelled at the beauty of where we live. Okay, so the grass needs cutting . . .

The next morning, I wake tired again. I do a body scan then walk down the road to Evandale Hair and Beauty for a buzz cut. Salon owner Sharyn Anderson asks how I've been travelling. I like Sharyn, who is cheerful and compassionate. I've been thinking about Soldier J and the support he said he got from his local community in country Victoria when he spoke openly about his PTSD.

Here goes. I tell Sharyn I just got out of a psych ward. Something about her reaction says she will understand, so I keep going, adding she is the first person in Evandale (apart from my family) who knows. She tells me about a policeman friend who she says manages his PTSD with meditation. I'm intrigued. Sharyn's friend, who I'll call Damian, texts me that night, inviting me to meet him at a Buddhist temple in Launceston in a couple of days.

The next day, Friday, I wake exhausted. Mary says I've run in my sleep almost every night since coming home. We drive into Launceston. I've booked a massage at a physiotherapy clinic because OT Michelle said, based on my sensory profile, massage would help. The therapist calls in sick. As I wait for Mary to pick me up after dropping the kids at school, a loud alarm from the nearby library shatters the relative calm. *Emergency! Evacuate!* I don't have my headphones. The alarm goes for ten minutes. *Stay calm. Breathe.*

At home, I go to bed and read *Dispatches*, Michael Herr's searing memoir of reporting on the Vietnam War. Herr covered the Tet Offensive, the Battle for Hue and the Siege of Khe Sanh. I was a wimp compared to the reporters in Vietnam.

I drag myself out of bed to pick Belle up from a school excursion. Our dog has left a pile of diarrhoea on the floor when we return. I'm teetering. It's another good excuse to go back to bed. Belle kindly cleans up after the dog. Then a gardener arrives to mow the lawn, which hasn't been cut in six weeks. My mower is busted. Because the grass is so long, he uses an industrial-sized brushcutter equipped with a three-pronged metal blade. The noise sounds like the American reconnaissance helicopters that flitted across Baghdad.

It's been a week since I left Ward 17. Is the honeymoon over? I'm isolating myself. I sense Mary is worried. The next morning, Saturday, I take Patrick to rowing training in Launceston. Heading home I worry I'll drive off the road, I'm so tired. I go back to bed. Damian sends me a text at 12.35 pm to say he is heading into the temple. The session doesn't start until 2 pm. On the way to Launceston, I stop at McDonalds for fries and a coke. At 1.20 pm I send myself an email: 'Is it possible to feel any more exhausted?' Maybe I mean depressed.

I find the temple, once an old Baptist church. It looks and feels like a Buddhist temple inside, with pictures of the Dalai

Lama, colourful wall hangings, flowers and statues. It smells of old wood. Damian shows me how to sit, lotus style. When it's time to meditate, just count your breaths, he says. A Lama (teacher) sits down, and we meditate for twenty minutes with eight other people. I count 226 breaths, a lot. I'll get down to 100–120 breaths over the coming weeks.

The Lama, originally from Tibet, says meditation takes time to master. The path to peace and happiness is not money, a big house or an important job. That equals stress. The answer is meditation. A couple of people ask questions and then he gets up and leaves. Energy flows through my body when I stand. I tell Damian that in the past I've never been able to focus like that during meditation. Without thinking, I say I'll attend 6 am meditation sessions at the temple each weekday.

At home, I collect some of the grass clippings left by the brush-cutter. I shower, then start rewriting my PTSD blog for Reuters. Mary is stunned at my transformation when she gets home. I tell her about the 6 am sessions. I'll come too, she says.

The next evening at 11 pm, I get up because I can't sleep and come out for some Valium. It's been a crazy day for all sorts of reasons. Mary is drinking a Corona in the living room. Let's start meditation on Tuesday, she says. Sounds good, I reply.

I assess how I'm doing against my Ward 17 discharge goals at the end of the following week. Lotus-style meditation has replaced body scans. I'm cooking and trying to reconnect with my family. I'm not practising good sleep hygiene. I haven't drunk rum, but I'm eating poorly. I haven't written my letter to Namir and Saeed. I miss my Ward 17 treating team and PTSD mates.

Thankfully, I have my first appointment with the psychologist recommended by Ward 17. I emailed him background on my admission and work history soon after my discharge. This appointment, this relationship, is crucial.

When we sit down, the psychologist says he hasn't read any of the material. He wants to hear everything from me. I can't believe it.

I persist for two more sessions. At one point he asks if I've told any clinician about all the trauma I've gone through. No, I say, not even in Ward 17, there wasn't time. I detect a sigh in his body language, like he's thinking, how did I get stuck with this loser? I cancel future appointments, saying we don't click.

My Ward 17 treating team warned me about setbacks, but I didn't expect it to be this rocky. Turns out this is normal after discharge from a psych ward. It makes sense. In Ward 17 everything was done for me: clinicians on hand, serenity, a place to think, mates who understood. Returning home was like getting off the plane in Jakarta: a burst of equatorial heat and the smell of kretek cigarettes, things I loved but an assault on the senses.

Truth is, I've come a long way from being suicidal two months ago. I'm getting my head around PTSD. I see a future myself. And there is a level of honesty with Mary that hasn't existed for a long time. Next challenge is getting back to work.

PART TWO

PART TWO

12

Rollercoaster

I resume work part-time in early October as planned, taking on my new role as a trainer and mentor for Reuters Asia. This is momentous on multiple levels. Patrick, Belle and Harry see their father at his desk again after seven months on sick leave. No matter how often I say I'm making progress, this proves it. It reassures Mary, who won't finish her Diploma in Community Services until mid-2017 and privately worries about the mortgage. And I need to show myself I'm still useful, even if I won't be doing journalism.

I haven't got a new contract, but I've had plenty of email exchanges and a lengthy discussion with HR about the role since it was first agreed in early July. Two days before my admission to Ward 17, the Asia boss called. I saw the name and considered letting it go to voicemail. I don't report to this person, but we've worked together for years. My direct manager arrived in Singapore not long after I went on sick leave. He hasn't called and never does.

I gritted my teeth and answered the only phone call I get from top editorial management in Singapore or New York all year. I'd sent emails to the bosses in Singapore during the previous five to six months, describing in detail my condition. I agonised over every word. In the first email, I said I was happy to talk on the phone and for colleagues to know what was going on. We should be open about mental illness, I wrote. But no one had sought to start a conversation with me about my treatment or my future. I agonised over every word in every email I sent and held my breath waiting for every response. Each one felt perfunctory. The emails said I was valued and so on. But it was akin to how my friend Jeremy Wagstaff described his meeting with the bosses. They had more important things to do.

To get a phone call two days before going to Ward 17 made me feel like I was a box being ticked.

The boss – whom I'm not going to identify – wished me good luck in Ward 17. I talked about the blogs, and mentoring and coaching young reporters when I was discharged. My blogs on PTSD could ease me back into work, the boss said, then asked me to help run a news leadership course in Singapore in November. The conversation was brief. 'Why did it take you so long to call?' I wanted to scream.

The next day, an HR executive reached out. I'd never spoken to this person before, whom I'll refer to by the gender-neutral name Reece, but I said I felt isolated at Reuters, lonely. I didn't plan to be so honest, it just happened. Reece sounded genuine, and texted me kind thoughts after I'd checked in to Ward 17 the following day.

Reece even visited me halfway through my admission. I showed Reece the ward and my room, then we had lunch at a nearby cafe. I hoped I had enough to offer Reuters despite being unable to return to my former role, I said. Reece insisted I did. Oh, the relief! Someone at Reuters believed I was worthy. With trust established, I said I'd been hospitalised because I was suicidal. I wanted to be honest. When I said my admission would exceed the maximum four weeks the boss had approved for payment, Reece said Reuters would cover the extra cost.

We talked about the blogs I planned to write, discussed my mentoring of young reporters and the training course in Singapore. Adjust to home life for two to three weeks before resuming work, Reece said, adding there was much I could do to also fix the company's program for supporting journalists with PTSD. I floated back into Ward 17, slid under my faded quilt, and slept. *I've finally found an ally.*

I'd entered Ward 17 with a job. Workers' comp wasn't grinding me into the dirt. I saw coppers forced to leave before they were ready because their insurer only paid for two weeks. Staff had one distressed copper in a wheelchair on Valium the night before her discharge. I wasn't a journalist anymore, but I still belonged to a global news organisation. I could put energy into my treatment.

The day after my discharge, Reece wished me well. I replied that I'd begin the blogs in early October as well as send a detailed outline on the mentoring role. The next step would be to come up with a loose plan of what the next few months looked like, Reece said, as well as get thoughts from the Asia boss.

Words and sentences poured onto my screen over the following days. The blogs become a 3000-word story that I hoped captured my journey from the Bali bombings to Ward 17.

On 3 October, I sent the story to the boss and Reece, saying Reuters could help break down the stigma of PTSD in the media industry by publishing it, not just circulating it internally.

Very few journalists anywhere have spoken publicly about struggling with PTSD. I emailed my blueprint on the mentoring role the same day. The boss said they would reply later with a more 'thoughtful' answer after recovering from the flu. In the meantime, the Singapore-based training editor was 'thrilled' to have me as co-coach for the November news leadership course, the boss said.

On 10 October, I began preparing slides on what a team of reporters needed to do to dominate a big story. I was getting into the groove of my new role.

Two days later, I call Reece about an issue with some PTSD expenses, which we quickly resolve. I'm keen for my story to be published, I say, adding it's the most important piece I've ever written. Reece says the editor-in-chief in New York will decide. That's fine, I reply. I'm ready to start mentoring, I just need the names of a few young reporters. I've not heard back about my blueprint, but figure I'll get started. I've mentored young journalists formally and informally since I was bureau chief in Vietnam in the late 1990s.

'We need to talk more about this role. Will it be permanent or not?' Reece says. It's the first time Reece has been business-like.

'What do you mean?' I ask.

'We don't have such a role globally. How long do we need a role like this?'

My body starts shaking. It knows where the conversation is headed. Reece is laying the groundwork to kill the new job.

Reuters wants a letter from my psychiatrist saying I can't do my current editing job, Reece says. I sent that months ago, I reply. I remind Reece that the Asia boss agreed in an email on 1 July – nearly three and a half months earlier – to the training and mentoring role. I have the email in front of me and read out the key bits.

'I need to talk to (the boss) about this,' Reece replies.

Gone is the warmth from Ward 17 and subsequent email exchanges. I'm shaking uncontrollably. My mouth is bone dry. It's hard to speak, but I get to the point.

'I feel like I'm fucked, like Reuters doesn't want me. If you want to get rid of me, just say so,' I say, my voice breaking.

Reece says nothing else of consequence but sends me a brief email an hour later in frightening HR language.

'What I understand from our conversation is that you do not want to nor cannot for health reasons return to your [editing] role. You have therefore submitted a proposal to perform a mentoring/coaching role for Reuters. In order for us to progress this it would be helpful to have documentation from your current treating psychiatrist stating you cannot perform your [editing] role due to your current injury. It will also be helpful for your psychiatrist to confirm that you are fit to return to work and to expand on capacity/duties you can perform on return – that may be the type of role, the number of hours, etc.'

I fill glass after glass with rum and coke and drink myself into a stupor and wake with a headache that lasts all day. The next night I cry out in my sleep. Mary says I was petrified, as if insurgents in Baghdad had finally caught me. I slip into a deep depression for days, powerless to stop what seems inevitable – getting thrown on the scrap heap.

Journal entry. Evandale, Oct 17, 2016: Feeling depressed. Today is going to be a struggle . . . went for a walk, see if I could snap out of it. Didn't work. Angry, depressed. Teary even but then I can't cry so what's the fucking point.

I'm trying to meditate when I wonder how many Valium and sleeping tablets I need for a fatal dose. I have plenty of both.

An email from Reece lands soon after. I'm in bed. Reuters wants to 'offer clarity' on the 'proposed' mentoring role.

'At the end of July you wrote to us expressing that you were not in a good way and that you wanted to be admitted to a facility. You requested the company pay for this treatment, which was agreed. You subsequently admitted yourself and stayed for 5 weeks. In our view at that time, the possibility of a mentoring role within the company was suspended indefinitely and it was expected that when you were well enough we would discuss with you an agreed return to work plan.'

The email reiterates that Reuters wants my treating psychiatrist to assess my capabilities against my existing editing duties, noting what I can and cannot do, or to talk to this person with my consent. Reuters had also notified its workers' compensation insurer, QBE Insurance, and was sending me documents to fill out. QBE would assist in managing 'my claim'. No claim had been discussed with me and the email gave no details, except to say I needed to complete paperwork for Reuters 'to progress this matter under the workers' compensation system'.

'We are committed to working with you to reach a positive outcome for you and for the business . . . We want to ensure that your return to work plan is conducive to your recovery and corresponds with the scope, pace and nature of work you are able to perform at this time and meets the needs and priorities of our business.'

I lie in bed for minutes, staring at the ceiling. Reuters knows I can't edit stories. It knows the only option is training/mentoring because I live in Tasmania. That means there is nothing I can do that meets the 'needs and priorities' of 'the business'. There is no return-to-work plan because there is no job.

They want me gone. They just don't have the guts to say so.

I send a profanity filled message to Jeremy who responds: 'Oh bollocks! That makes no sense chronology wise.'

Energised with rage, I fling the doona off and get up.

Three hours later, the general manager for Southeast Asia emails, giving me approval to travel to Singapore for the November training course. HR and whoever else is involved in this attempt to drive me out forget to tell him.

When I realised months earlier that I couldn't do news anymore, I sought advice from an employment lawyer in Hobart about the implications for my contract with Reuters. Those concerns were allayed when Reuters agreed to the training and mentoring job. A couple of days after being told that role had been abolished, I call the same lawyer who says her initial assessment is that a contract exists over it given the detail and frequency of discussions even though nothing was signed. But she suggests my complaint is more about personal injury and how Reuters failed to properly support me after I was diagnosed with PTSD. She's right – to me, that is far more important.

I call Cait McMahon from the Dart Center for Journalism and Trauma, who gives me the name of Bree Knoester, managing partner of AdviceLine Injury Lawyers in Melbourne (now principal lawyer with Brave Legal). Bree represented photographer AZ, who lost her case against *The Age* in 2013 and who I wanted to visit while in Ward 17. I make an appointment to see Bree in Melbourne the following week.

When a case manager from QBE calls, I tell her a mistake has been made, I *can* work, I want nothing to do with workers' comp.

*

A few days later, I'm stunned to be told senior editors in New York want to publish my PTSD blog as a Reuters special report. It's a decision that will save my career, and halt the mental spiral I've been on.

Mike Williams, the global enterprise editor based in New York, emails me: 'I read [your story] on the ferry across the Hudson River to work the other day, and by the time the boat landed, tears were streaming down my cheeks.'

Mike is one of the best long-form journalism editors in the world and previously held senior positions at the *Wall Street Journal*. Some Reuters colleagues think he's blunt and uncompromising, but I like him. I didn't know Mike had the piece. That's a surprise itself. His reaction is even more unexpected. *My story made him cry yet I'm unmoved.*

Special reports are multimedia packages of text, pictures, TV and graphics, usually published on a microsite. Not many Reuters journalists get special reports published. They take months to prepare and edit. The pitching process is exhaustive and the rejection rate high. My first instinct is to ignore Mike. I suspect he knows nothing about what's going on in Asia (he doesn't), but either way, I'm still taking legal action, I tell Jeremy. I'm too angry, the betrayal is too deep. And I'll offer my story to the *New York Times* or *The Guardian* if it's that good. Jeremy tries to reason with me, but I brush him off.

Mary insists I reply positively to Mike. 'You made him cry!' she says.

'You don't understand,' I shout. 'They drew the line in the sand and there is no going back!'

'Because I love you so much, I want you to think about this,' Mary replies gently. 'Ask people in New York if they were aware of the HR email.'

I pause.

'Jeremy says I should be cautious too.'

'See, please listen to us. You're not thinking straight, which is understandable,' Mary says.

I could have killed myself over that email from HR, I tell her, burying my face in my hands at the magnitude of those words. Mary moves closer, puts her arm around my back. We are sitting on the couch in the living room.

Something, maybe Mary's touch, her softness, gets me to see sense. She and Jeremy are right. Maybe there is a better way to resolve things over the story, I say. But I can't keep working for Reuters. The betrayal is too deep.

I used to think I felt such betrayal because I could have been killed working for Reuters in Baghdad. That was validated when I met veterans and coppers in Ward 17. Similar situations. What I'll come to realise is that this betrayal – this form of moral injury – can affect anyone if their notion of 'what's right' has been violated strongly enough. I know because enough people have told me their stories. And they've never been near a warzone. But their organisations, the justice system, the government, treated them like lepers.

It was more than the physical risks I took. I *did* give my life to Reuters. I gave them *everything*, the way I covered stories, the hours I put in, and my family and I paid the price. I expected the organisation to look after me, not try to force me out.

Jeremy and I once discussed how the problem might have been a lack of manager training in Asia. I'll later find a video message announcing the establishment of the Reuters peer network in mid-2015. In it, the editor-in-chief says: 'Our managers continue to receive training to understand how traumatic events affect us and how to respond.' On the company's internal website, I'll see an e-learning trauma support module that says to managers:

'If you send someone on leave, offer to stay in touch so that they do not become isolated.' It's like a cruel joke.

'Would you really have killed yourself?' Mary asks quietly.

I think. 'No, what I meant was it was a situation in which someone might have. I was too angry to do so.'

After my discharge from Ward 17, I'd promised Mary to tell her if I felt suicidal. In our living room now, I say I'll never take my life, leave my family. I have too much to live for, too much to do. Nevertheless, Mary prays she won't find me dead each time she gets home from TAFE.

I wake at 3 am the following morning, 26 October. I'm due to fly to Melbourne to see Bree. My two sleeping tablets have worn off. I lie in bed thinking, then run Mary through scenarios when we get up: do the special report, quit Reuters, negotiate a payout and start a new life.

Mary suggests I call Alix Freedman, the company's global head of ethics and standards. A Pulitzer Prize–winning journalist, Alix is the final reader on signature stories, especially sensitive ones. She also works closely with Mike on special reports. Like Mike, I respect Alix. I've had her pick apart a few pieces I've edited over the years that didn't meet her standards. I call. Alix read my PTSD story before Mike.

'I usually hate first-person journalism, but I loved, loved, loved this,' she tells me from New York. 'I said to Mike, I want you to read this story. I didn't give him any background, I just said, read it. If we got copy like this all the time I'd have fewer grey hairs.'

Alix is unaware of what HR in Asia is doing until I tell her, but says I should 'kick that can down the road'. She adds, 'You have a spectacular story here. Let's get it organised.'

I've gotten sky-high praise from two of the toughest editors not just at Reuters, anywhere. It barely registers. All that matters to me is the betrayal. In Melbourne, while waiting to see Bree at her office, I make some notes. Maybe Mary is right. Maybe I'm being too hasty:

- *Do special report. Possibly a follow-up piece.*
- *Those responsible for the Oct 17 email must be held accountable.*
- *Fix Reuters' PTSD program (perhaps).*
- *Quit Reuters. Negotiate payout, nothing that muzzles me. Psych bills covered for life.*
- *Write a book.*
- *New career. PTSD advocacy, writer, public speaker, change policy.*
- *Don't want mentoring role. Something has broken inside me.*

I meet Bree and one of her colleagues, an employment law expert. Bree has been a solicitor and barrister for nearly fifteen years, representing ordinary people in some of Victoria's largest compensation cases. Bree says the key issue with duty of care is whether Reuters adequately prepared me for the potential psychological damage of covering the Iraq War, the Boxing Day tsunami and the Bali bombings. No, they didn't, I reply. I did a five-day hostile environment course in Britain in 2001 but that was about first-aid, spotting minefields, getting through fake checkpoints – physical safety. Reuters also set up a 24/7 trauma support hotline in 2006. I used it after Namir and Saeed were killed. Bree says media organisations had been on notice about the importance of peer support networks since 2002, when the BBC established one. Reuters didn't follow suit until 2015.

But all my editors were supportive when I was in the field, especially as Baghdad bureau chief, I say. They had my back. I'm not dragging them into this.

Bree's colleague, the employment lawyer, reckons I could successfully sue Reuters for breach of contract over the training/mentoring role but only get a year's salary and be gagged in a settlement.

I slump back in a leather chair, deflated. I've got no legal moves to make. It would be immoral to accuse my old editors of negligence when I wanted those tough assignments. I never asked to be taken off a story or said my mental health was suffering. They all regularly checked on me, cared about me. It's the bosses in Singapore and New York I want held accountable. The understanding of journalist trauma has grown so much in the past decade.

Back home in Evandale, I contact the global head of HR in New York, who I've never spoken to before, asking if we can discuss the 17 October email. I've cancelled the Singapore trip and ignored emails and phone messages from Reece, including one suggesting there might have been a misunderstanding. The head of HR, who has read my story, replies: 'I want you to know that your contributions to Reuters are vast and very important to us and we would all like that to continue.'

Maybe I still have a future at Reuters.

The email was worded poorly, the global head of HR tells me on the phone. After being prepped by Mary and Jeremy to be professional, I leave it at that.

'Let's talk about the training and mentoring role,' the HR chief says.

'I'm not interested in that now,' I reply.

It's been 26 days since I'd got an email that was intended to force me to quit or put me in the ghastly worker's compensation system – Bree and the employment lawyer in Tasmania agreed they were the likely scenarios. The chilling abandonment and loss of identity I'd seen among veterans and coppers in Ward 17 was to be my fate. I'd drawn up a list of possible occupations outside Reuters. In my current state of mind, not long out of a psych ward, the future looked grim. Who would hire me?

I've been forced to think deeply about my future, I tell the head of HR. I want to become a PTSD advocate for Reuters. There is momentary silence, but to my surprise, she likes the idea. I send her a proposal that revolves around me improving the company's trauma support program and writing a manual on PTSD for staff and managers, including what editors should do when a journalist is diagnosed. I don't want colleagues to experience what I have. Dr Maryam writes a letter saying the role would give me purpose and assist in my recovery, adding I must take it slowly.

—

I'm anxious the day before Reuters publishes my special report. I worry about the impact on my family. Mary and I have told the kids we want to raise awareness of PTSD, encourage others to be open about mental illness. I brace for criticism for drawing attention to myself when others were more stoic or worse off. I expect negative comments from those who hate WikiLeaks or criticism of the US military. I'm also hoping the story will have a positive impact, help people.

The special report is headlined *The Road to Ward 17: My battle with PTSD*. It includes a podcast, photographs, a snippet of the Collateral Murder tape and a graphic. The story is published in the early hours of 15 November, Evandale time. As usual, my sleeping tablets wear off about 3 am. I check my phone from bed.

My email inbox is filling up with beautiful messages. I get up and turn on my laptop. Colleagues and friends from the United States are putting the story on Facebook, which I rejoined recently to be part of a group of Ward 17 patients after a years-long absence. The positive reaction, the outpouring of support, floors me. I belong to that breed of journalist who just covered the news. The story was never about us.

Hundreds of people from around the world will tell me the story resonated with them. Many are strangers. A nun in New York. The wife of a Vietnam veteran with PTSD. A therapist in Lisbon. A mother whose journalist son is returning to the United States after ten years working in the Middle East. Those and many ordinary people write to me of their trauma – the death of a child, the suicide of a loved one, child abuse, sexual assault. Guilt and shame are common threads. Scores of journalists thank me for speaking out on an issue many have struggled with in silence. I've opened a collective wound.

Copper Matt Ross calls: 'Mate, keep writing because you can put into words stuff that we don't know how to.'

A couple of days after the story is published, I post this comment on Facebook: 'I've had a lot of people tell me how brave I've been to share my story. To me, the real brave people are the men and women I met in Ward 17 – military veterans, coppers and emergency service folks – who showed enormous strength despite everything thrown at them. Dealing with PTSD is tough enough, but I haven't had to battle with insurance companies about my diagnosis (yet) or struggle for a decent compensation payout or find another job. I haven't had to struggle with addiction, apart from a couple of months where I couldn't get through the day without plenty of rum and coke . . . Everyone's support has meant so much to me.'

At the same time, I tell Jeremy I feel like I'm drowning in a sea of trauma.

Journal entry. Evandale, Nov 18, 2016: It's hard to describe my feelings to what has happened since the story was published. There is so much pain out there, and guilt and loss.

It takes weeks to reply to the emails and Facebook messages. I hope that in some small way my story will help drive a public debate around the need to better understand PTSD and break the stigma and prejudice surrounding it. I do interviews with media in Australia and the United States, which spur more messages.

Journal entry. Evandale, Nov 21, 2016. Just hanging on to my sanity. So much to do. So many emails to respond to.

What I've done – though I don't understand this nor realise its importance yet – is communalise my trauma. I've shared my story and people from all walks of life have listened and embraced me. But I've gone out the gate too fast. Before I'm well enough.

In early December, Mary says I'm sleeping poorly, running in my sleep. One night I cry out. Unprocessed memories keep me in bed or force me under the covers sometimes during the day. I've stopped meditating and walking. The emails and Facebook messages keep coming.

I make a list.

– *Emails to answer.*
– *Establish an independent website about PTSD for journalists with Matthew Green, a former Reuters colleague I worked with in Baghdad who lives in London.*

- *Get local companies to sponsor two Melbourne women running marathons across Tasmania to raise money for mental health charities.*
- *Sort out a plan with Soldier D, my mate from Ward 17, to walk the Overland Track in Tasmania to raise money for charity.*
- *Help organise a trivia night in Evandale to raise money for another veteran who trains PTSD service dogs.*

I've also been thinking about follow-up stories to the special report. One is to try to track down the pilots of Crazy Horse 1–8. They've never been far from my mind these past six months.

—

I contact a former medic from the 2nd Battalion, 16th Infantry Regiment, Michael 'Doc' Bailey, who was at the scene after Namir and Saeed were killed. Michael treated the only adult to survive. The battalion's senior medic looked after the two wounded children of minivan driver Saleh Matasher Tomal. Michael is active on Facebook and happy to chat. We have two long, amiable phone conversations. Employed by Home Depot now, America's equivalent to Bunnings, Michael sounds tired and unfulfilled in civilian life. Fourteen of the roughly 800 men in the 2–16 were killed during their fifteen-month deployment to Baghdad. At 33, Michael remembers dead comrades and maimed Iraqi kids.

Rules of engagement didn't just apply to combat. Michael often argued with his lieutenant because he wanted to take wounded Iraqis to American hospitals. His LT wouldn't budge. The ROEs said no, unless US soldiers or ordnance were the cause.

Before Michael's unit left their base at dawn on 12 July 2007, the day Namir and Saeed were killed, mortars rained down and soldiers took cover, he recalls. Firefights broke out across al-Amin that morning. I ask Michael why the Iraqi men Namir and Saeed were with walked about so casually. It was their territory, they knew where we were, Michael replies.

'If you watch the video, you can see what's going on in their minds in the way they move. They weren't concerned. We were in their area. They were going to ambush us.'

What they didn't consider were the two Apache gunships.

Michael was diagnosed with PTSD the following year and in 2009 tried to suicide twice before the military tossed him out of the army. 'They fucked me hardcore,' he says. Still, he misses the life, the camaraderie.

'There is a sense of purpose that comes with putting the uniform on that I don't have anymore, a sense of worth I have from my combat medical badge that civilians don't appreciate.'

Michael hates Collateral Murder. He started a Facebook group for 2–16 veterans after the video was released.

'I'll be honest, at the time I didn't feel much sympathy for your photographer. I thought what he did was stupid, he walked right into that. Years later, I realised I needed to show more compassion, he was focused on his job, he didn't know he was in danger . . . As a medic I put myself in a lot of danger. I just went to my guys and treated them.'

Michael and I haven't agreed on everything, but we find common humanity, two men with PTSD on opposite sides of the world bound by one day in Baghdad. He suggests I contact one of his Facebook friends, a former Apache pilot who flew in the same unit as the Crazy Horse 1–8 crew. This man vigorously defended them after Collateral Murder was published. I send this man, who I'll refer to as Dan, a message saying I want to talk to the pilots. I'm not seeking retribution. I just want to know how everything has affected them.

Dan says he'll forward my message, but doesn't think they will respond. 'Knowing the kind of things these guys and their families have put up with since that tape came out, I seriously doubt they will talk. I'm sorry you're suffering. It's understandable you feel at least partially responsible for the loss of people working for you . . . I hope you can find peace. Having seen the entire tape several times, if I had been there that day, I would have pulled the trigger myself. The weapons were easily identifiable, and they were in an area where U.S. ground forces had been taking fire.'

I tell Dan I'll fly to the United States to meet the pilots, try to get to know them. The time for remonstration and anger had passed. It's time to heal, I say.

'I think it could help the healing for many people involved on many levels if I was to write about such a coming together. I would guarantee their anonymity, in writing.'

Journal entry. Evandale, Dec 2016: Why do I want to talk to the pilots? I genuinely want to know how they feel. I won't deny it could make for a good story, especially if they talk in person. But there is a bigger issue here – how we atone for our perceived wrongdoing or failure in war or other situations. It's about how we heal. It's about setting an example for others to follow. If the pilots are suffering, I want to help them. I'm suffering, I'd like to think they could help me too. It won't happen if all those involved in that dreadful day don't tell their stories.

Dan goes quiet for a while. He apologises when I chase him up, saying he's only kept in touch with two of the four men in the air that day. He doesn't say which ones. I'd assumed both were from Crazy Horse 1–8. They might have been. Dan says one understood my desire to talk but wanted to put the event behind him. He got no reply from the other.

One evening a few days before Christmas, I drive to a community radio station in Launceston for an interview with Jo Fidgen from the BBC *Outlook* program in London. Jo kindly asks if anything is off limits over the next hour. No, I reply. She gets me with her first question, asking me to paint the scene at the Bali bombings and how I felt. My heart starts racing. Bali has affected me more than I thought. Jo moves to Aceh, asks me to describe difficult images. I mention the burnt girl on the stretcher and a child covered with cardboard.

We talk about Iraq, and for the first time in months I struggle to explain what happened to Namir and Saeed. I can't stitch the narrative together. *What is wrong with me?* I wave my arms about in this tiny studio as if that might help, even though Jo can't see me. 'What do you mean you were responsible?' Jo keeps asking. I need to atone, I plan to write Namir and Saeed a letter, I reply.

Jo catches me off-guard by asking if I've written a similar letter to Mary. *How does she know?* I have, but it's too personal to discuss on air, I say.

Then Jo wants to know why I went to Ward 17. I try to spell it out, without saying suicide. She gets it in the end. I've done several lengthy media interviews since my special report was published and felt okay. But this is different. I'm sweaty and exhausted, prised open, which is not Jo's fault. She feels awful when I tell her. No, I said go for it.

Back home, I tell Mary it was tough going. We don't talk much but the next morning I find her in the garden, so upset she can barely speak. Mary had been getting worried about everything I'd taken on and tried to warn me. The interview made me understand I need to focus on my recovery, I say as if I've had a revelation.

'I've been trying to tell you this,' Mary says. 'You've become manic about helping others and not yourself. If *you* recover, so will the kids and me. You're using all these projects to avoid processing your trauma.'

'No, these projects are meaningful, I get meaning from them,' I say.

Then it dawns on me. It is avoidance. Mary is right.

'The folks at Ward 17 were worried I'd get manic. How did I forget this?'

———

About a month after I came home from Ward 17, I was doing my morning walk in Evandale. The sun was shining. I was thinking about Soldier D and his plan to do the Overland Track. I said I'd go along, get him media interviews, do a Facebook campaign for his fundraising efforts.

For some reason, I pictured Soldier D and I hiking up to the old miner's hut in the Tarkine. Tears welled in my eyes. I couldn't believe it. I was crying. I looked around to see if anyone was watching as I strode around the village oval. Then I thought, *Fuck, let it go*. And I did, two full laps, including sitting on a wooden bench seat with my head in my hands. *Thank God, I can feel emotion*. Images of Namir and Saeed popped into my mind. Then I went back to thinking about Soldier D. The strength of the man. His determination to help others.

Soldier D and two other Ward 17 mates come for lunch a few days after Christmas. One is a former copper from the nearby town of Longford. The other a veteran from Devonport. Soldier D has been seeing his mum in Queenstown and is going back to Ward 17 for another admission. Like many veterans with PTSD I've met, Soldier D seems directionless. He's on so much medication he can't drive trucks, the only full-time job he's had since the army discharged him. He lives outside Canberra, getting occasional work chopping firewood, but little else. His purpose in life comes by hiking long distances to raise money for veteran's charities.

'Mate, I can't help with the Overland Track,' I say.

'No worries,' he replies.

You never have to explain yourself to someone with PTSD.

Soldier D is on fire over lunch, telling great stories. But he looks shaky.

After my friends leave, Mary and I sit outside. Her favourite cat Mas Biru emerges from under a hedge, ambles over for a scratch. The water in the South Esk River is low enough to walk across. Mary says she sensed I wanted to go with Soldier D back to Ward 17. A part of me did: the routine. Walk, write, therapy, sleep. I crave that simple life.

13

Psychs who really *see* me

By early 2017, discussions about becoming the Reuters PTSD advocate are going well with New York. I've withdrawn from some of the mental health side-projects I'd been involved in. Mary gets a job counselling refugees and asylum seekers – casualties of the wars in Afghanistan and Iraq and conflict in Sri Lanka, Eritrea, South Sudan and Ethiopia.

Some balance is returning to my life, although I'm still struggling with headaches and fatigue. I sleep a few hours every second afternoon. I also sense unprocessed trauma from my nightmares. In one, waves surge along the South Esk River. From my backyard, I watch a yellow ute try to outrun the torrent. It's probably the farmer who checks his sheep and cattle grazing near the bank. I'm not sure if he makes it. In another nightmare, staff at Ward 17 try to kill me when I arrive for admission, thinking I'm sneaking in to do a story. In yet another, bandits are beheading people on the roadside as I drive to Moscow to cover a city on the brink.

*

I still haven't written my letter to Namir and Saeed.

In between shit days, I have amazing ones. Mary's eyes widen when I tell her Reuters has nominated my special report for a Pulitzer Prize in feature writing. I'm honoured and humbled. I get an email from three filmmakers in Sydney who are developing a documentary on PTSD and first responders. After reading my special report they want me to narrate the film. I'm blown away by the opportunity to do something so meaningful.

Mary decides it's time to tell me things I didn't know: how each night for years she put on a happy face because she knew I was struggling, even though I wouldn't admit I had PTSD; that she'd been drinking at home in Singapore and Evandale at night after I'd gone to bed in despair over my angry outbursts, worried whether our marriage could be repaired, and how she might start over with three young children; that after she dropped me at the airport to fly to Ward 17 she wept. She tried so hard to keep the family together, to protect the children from my anger, but to also shield me from the rambunctious twists and turns of family life and the animals that brought them joy and comfort. She'd had to be everywhere but found herself nowhere.

The therapy I did in Ward 17 has allowed us to dig deeper. Ever the journalist, Mary asks probing questions, often as we walk around Evandale on weekends. This has unintended consequences. It has at times triggered memories of her own traumatic experiences as a journalist.

One morning in late December 2016, I could tell Mary was upset. We were sitting in the kitchen. She told me about a girl with spina bifida she had seen in central Vietnam in the late 1990s, locked in a dark shed each day when her parents went to the rice fields. The girl was about seven or eight. Central Vietnam was a key battlefield of the war. Mary said she was horrified she'd done nothing to help the girl. We talked through her options: inform local authorities? Give the parents money so they could have paid someone to look after their daughter? The first option would have been ignored or landed the family in trouble. Would it have helped the girl? No. In the second option, the parents would have used the cash to buy necessities. But the girl still would have been locked up.

On that same trip, Mary came across a boy who was slowly starving to death because of shrapnel embedded in his jaws. He'd been playing in nearby fields when he detonated a piece of unexploded ordnance. Again, Mary said she had done nothing. Could she have gotten the boy surgery, outside Vietnam perhaps? She was racked with guilt.

I told Mary I suspected this was her own moral injury. We talked about things that might help her. Visit Vietnam. Donate money to a charity. Write about her experiences. We noted other journalists would be haunted by similar memories. Mary said this had given her an insight into my moral injury and that she would surely feel better the next day. She did, though the relief was temporary.

Another time, Mary confided, her self-confidence dropped when she stopped working in 2001 to have our children, when she no longer earned money. We were living in Jakarta, where Reuters paid me a tax-free salary and provided our housing, so financially we were secure. But like me, journalism was integral to Mary's identity. Suddenly, she had three toddlers on her hands within three years, and I was hardly home. Mary worried about being a good mother. She was tired, felt insecure about her body. She miscarried in 2006. Her superannuation balance is only 10 per cent of mine.

Mary wonders why I still find her attractive.

'Because you are a beautiful woman, a beautiful person,' I say.

'We need to work on our intimacy,' Mary says.

'I just want to start kissing again. I love it when we spoon in bed,' I reply.

I feel a warm glow between us. Mary is my rock.

We reminisce about our early years. Our tiny flat in Hong Kong, eating out nearly every night, the old Kai Tak airport just a short taxi ride away to destinations across Asia and beyond. Me hiring an old Mercedes taxi in Cairo to pick Mary up from the airport after I'd arrived a day earlier from backpacking around Syria. Mary soaking in a bath for ages, enjoying all the oils $1000 a night got in the Shangri-La Hotel in Hong Kong, while I paced outside waiting to propose. Hong Kong and its harbour were ablaze with neon from celebrations to mark Britain's transfer of power back to China a few days earlier. Mary and I riding bicycles to work in Hanoi, braving the cyclos and new Honda motorbikes. Tucking into steaming bowls of pho, delicious soup served from big vats for breakfast. Drinking homemade beer on tiny plastic stools in late afternoon on the pavement.

Journal entry. Evandale, Jan 26, 2017: I have a loving wife who understands me, who is on this journey with me. We make so much progress in our talks, get to the bottom of things. Sometimes, on many days, however, it's fucking hard. The urge to go back to bed so strong, to feed my face with chocolate and ice cream. That depressive cloak so tight.

—

In mid-February 2017 I wonder if I've reached a turning point. Good days outnumber the bad. If I get up early and walk, then meditate and write for an hour or two, the day usually goes well. The challenge is to manage everything.

I'm also about to see a psychologist called Wendy Gall in Launceston. Wendy was recommended by a nurse I know who developed PTSD after working in North Africa for Médecins Sans Frontières (MSF). This will be my first therapy since leaving Ward 17 five months ago. The psychologist I saw after my discharge doesn't count.

I'd emailed Wendy at the end of 2016 asking if she was taking new clients. I included a link to my special report and other media interviews I'd done. I told Wendy I wanted to explore ways to deal with my moral injury, such as modifying the Adaptive Disclosure program to fit my situation. By then I'd pored over the book *Adaptive Disclosure: A New Treatment for Military Trauma, Loss and Moral Injury* by Brett Litz and his co-authors Leslie Lebowitz, Matt Gray and William Nash. Lebowitz is a clinical psychologist who did trauma training for the US military; Gray a professor of psychology at the University of Wyoming, whose research has focused on the emotional and psychological impact of combat; Nash is director of psychological health for the US Marine Corps.

I'd also emailed Litz, asking if he thought moral injury could apply to journalists and if so, would Adaptive Disclosure be appropriate treatment. Litz said he and his colleagues never intended their work to be exclusive to the military. While he didn't fully comprehend all the conflicts and challenges journalists faced, he was sure moral injury was a risk for my profession. 'I would assume that threats to personal safety on the job can be traumatizing for some, especially if they are acute and unprecedented,' Litz wrote. 'However, I would assume most journalists would be more haunted and impacted by being exposed to violence as an observer in real-time or bearing witness to violence and cruelty. The outcome would not be a racing heart in the sense of phobias and PTSD from life-threat, but more akin to a broken heart.'

Litz nailed it. I know many journalists with PTSD who I suspect are imprisoned in the moral dimension of their experiences. The horror. The injustice. A sense their work hasn't made any difference. Ask any journalist who reported from the Middle East. It broke their hearts.

Litz said he assumed some journalists could also experience 'high stakes' betrayal from their organisation or local decision-makers when their lives were at risk or peers died.

Adaptive Disclosure could 'quite possibly' be used to treat journalists, but this would have to be answered scientifically. Adaptive Disclosure was developed with the military culture in mind, and would need adjusting for the culture and context journalists worked in. But the basic elements of treatment would be the same, he added.

That was good enough for me.

Wendy was taking January off but could see me in February. The links I sent gave her 'great background', she said, so I ordered her the Adaptive Disclosure book and dropped it at her office while she was on leave. I'd like to try a customised version if you're game, I said in another email.

Adaptive Disclosure attempts to help veterans accept what they did or didn't do without minimising culpability. Techniques include the sharing of stories with a therapist or chaplain, getting encouragement from peers, and writing letters, sometimes apologising to the person they believe they wronged. Veterans don't have to send the letters, but it helps them move forward. The goal, say Litz and his colleagues, is to foster balance and acceptance, as well as reclaim goodness. They believe cognitive behaviour therapy (CBT), for example, might not work with moral injury because a clinician will likely challenge a patient's view of their culpability, saying it's negative or distorted thinking. Many journalists and others – even to this day – tell me I wrongly blamed myself over Namir and Saeed's deaths. This misses a point that I suspect only someone who has been in a similar situation can understand, which is this: I know what I could have done. I didn't live up to the expectations I set for myself. I must own that and work through it.

Wendy said she would skim the book before she saw me.

I know by now that it's vital to have a good rapport with your clinician. American psychiatrist Bessel van der Kolk says a patient must feel comfortable with their therapist to the point of having 'deep positive feelings' for them. The therapist must engage with the patient too, he writes in his best-selling 2014 book, *The Body Keeps the Score: Brain, Mind and Body in the Healing of Trauma*.

'The critical question is this: Do you feel that your therapist is curious to find out who you are and what you, not some generic "PTSD patient", need? Are you just a list of symptoms on some diagnostic questionnaire, or does your therapist take the time to find out why you do what you do and think what you think?' van der Kolk said.

Dr Maryam exemplified what van der Kolk writes about. By reading the links I sent her, so did Wendy. She validated my story. She was effectively saying, *I see you, Dean*. Her willingness to consider trying something out of left field showed she respected my understanding of my trauma and gave me a sense of control over the process.

*

Wendy and I sit opposite each other in her tidy office in Launceston. She rests a large notepad on her lap. I thank her for taking the time to review the material I sent. Wendy has been a psychologist for about 25 years, making us roughly the same age. She likes to help people manage their condition or circumstances and come to terms with what happened, she says. While Wendy doesn't consider herself an expert on PTSD, some of her clients have been badly traumatised. She wants to get to know me over two or three sessions, then see if we can use Adaptive Disclosure based on her understanding of my needs and the treatment model, which makes sense.

After I talk about my childhood, Mary and the kids, Wendy says, 'Okay, what's bothering you right now?' My brain goes blank then into hyperdrive. Right foot tapping, I reel off how I only recently grasped the depth of my trauma over the Bali bombings; I describe my bodily sensations during the BBC interview with Jo Fidgen; the pain in some of the messages I got after my special report was published, the stories people shared with me; how I'm avoiding the processing I need to do; even whether my suicidal thoughts were real.

The floodgates are open.

I'm only beginning to grasp the pressure I was under running the Baghdad bureau during the Iraq War; I haven't watched Collateral Murder, haven't written to Namir and Saeed. I also throw in my new role at Reuters and the documentary.

Wendy doesn't interrupt much. I think she understands that after no therapy in five months, I have a lot to say. She draws a line across a blank piece of paper, then writes *extreme* and *minimal* at either end.

'First impressions,' she says. 'There is a lot going on in your head, and some confusion too.' She says I got a bit manic as I spoke, which concerned her.

'You bounced between both ends of this line. You struggled to comprehend you had suicidal thoughts even though Maryam reassured you about this. You questioned how you could get PTSD, saying you weren't shot at or blown up, but then you described a series of experiences that were clearly traumatic.'

At the end of our session, Wendy says I might feel tired later. I vomit for several hours that evening. Mary considers taking me to emergency at Launceston General Hospital. The next morning, I'm washed out and sleep in the afternoon, then I get a headache that lasts all night.

Journal Entry. Evandale, Feb 15, 2017. My physical reaction of the past 36 hours is a bit frightening. It would be so easy to forget the therapy if it's going to be this difficult. Just roll on . . . Wouldn't it be easier to push everything to the back of my mind? Not sure I understand what is going on.

—

The documentary filmmakers want to move fast. They need to make a trailer to present to film bodies and broadcasters to raise funds for full production. At the end of March, two of the filmmakers, Helen Barrow and Susan Lambert, fly to Evandale for a couple of days. They do separate interviews with Mary and myself as well as film me in the rainforest. Everything goes smoothly, I'm on home soil. But next up is a visit to Ward 17 and then a conference on the mental health of first responders in Melbourne.

I can't sleep the night before we fly out. I wake anxious and agitated. I'm even dizzy, which rarely happens. I have no idea why. I calm down when we get to Melbourne. I'm in journalist mode, I have a job to do.

Helen films me walking through the glass door of Ward 17, then heading to the medical room to sit in the chair where my vital signs were taken each day. I'm not pretending to look pensive, it's real. Back in the corridor, I see social worker Christina Sim, who gives me a big hug, then it's off to interview Maryam in the group meeting room.

I've looked forward to this since the filmmakers suggested visiting Ward 17. Maryam and I smile and shake hands. It's okay to hug my social worker, not my psychiatrist. Maryam is several months pregnant with her first child. I'm delighted for her.

'I can't believe I'm here,' I say, as Helen clips a mic onto Maryam.

'What do you mean?' Maryam asks.

'It was when we arrived, seeing Ward 17, it felt like yesterday. I think it's because Ward 17 is so important to me,' I say. I describe my body over the past 24 hours. My mind has been fine, it's my body. Maryam corrects me: It's your mind *and* your body, the conversation between them.

I recall when Maryam told me Ward 17 was an introduction to treatment, how I'd blocked the reality of the long road ahead.

'I always talk about the process, or the journey,' Maryam says. 'The first step is having an understanding, an insight into what is happening and then feeling the need for treatment, help-seeking, whatever you want to call it. People need to understand this process can take a long time.'

I'm supposed to ask Maryam about first responders, but I can't help myself. I'm sitting in front of a psychiatrist who gets me, who listened, who wanted to hear my story the moment we met six months ago.

'Why do you think I can't write my letter to Namir and Saeed?'

'It might be avoidance, you might not be ready,' Maryam replies.

'Did it make sense why I wanted to watch Collateral Murder?'

'Of course,' Maryam says. 'Most people either have huge gaps in their memory of a traumatic event or they remember a lot of detail.'

Then she hits me with a major revelation, which I don't have time to reflect on just yet.

'You wanted to fill in the gaps because I think being shown those first few minutes of footage in Baghdad was the most traumatising moment of your career.'

'Remember we also spoke about survivor's guilt?' adds Maryam. 'There are people who live with this as part of their PTSD. They might go back and recheck a thousand times in their mind to see what could have been done differently but they have no footage. In your case you did. It's not always logical. It's about your emotions. Emotionally I think you wanted to go back and see what could have been done differently.'

'What about me going to Baghdad?'

'It's a risk. Any triggers that remind you of the trauma can exacerbate PTSD. Going back to the exposure scene is going to expose you to things that happened. Is it a good idea? I think that will depend on your mental health at the time.'

'But I have to atone, come to some sort of acceptance over what happened.'

'That's why I am not saying yes or no . . . We've had Vietnam veterans go back to Vietnam. Some even live there. So, it's not impossible for people to go back to the scene of their trauma.'

Helen, who is filming, whispers in my ear to ask about first responders.

I ask Maryam if society understands the impact trauma has on police and emergency service personnel. She says while first responders are trained and know the risks, many people forget they are human beings who go home to partners and children.

'I don't think we quite get it if we don't see it happen, don't see the consequences,' Maryam says. 'If I wasn't a psychiatrist working here I might think it's their job. They are meant to do this. But there are limits and there is always baggage we carry from our personal lives.'

'What about first responders with PTSD getting back to work, when it's vital to their identity?'

Maryam says she spoke to a patient yesterday about this.

'Often, we've got people here who are second, third and fourth generation veterans or police. It's their heritage, their identity, it's their life . . . I remember we talked a lot about Viktor Frankl and the meaning of life. To lose their job is a big loss.'

'So how can you recover when something is so important to you?' I ask.

'It's essential to define what recovery means,' Maryam replies. Veterans and police with PTSD are generally looking for meaning in life. She says many veterans find this by advocating for other vets. It's possible for first responders with PTSD to return to previous roles, but care needs to be taken because they have risky jobs and high expectations of themselves.

I could interview Maryam all day, but we have another appointment. It's been wonderful seeing her. I wish her well with the birth of her child.

We pack up and leave Ward 17. Helen drives to the Florey Institute of Neuroscience and Mental Health, twenty minutes away. I'm due to interview Professor Alexander 'Sandy' McFarlane, director of the Centre for Traumatic Stress Studies (CTSS) at the University of Adelaide. Professor McFarlane, a psychiatrist, is respected around the world for his research into PTSD and the treatment of sufferers, often in military and natural disaster contexts. In a landmark study in 2000, he showed how traumatised people couldn't filter and analyse information properly. Key parts of their brains failed them.

I start to feel nauseated in the car. At the Florey Institute I lie on a couch while we wait for the professor. I want to throw up. Helen is both concerned and curious. She suggests I ask him if my visit to Ward 17 has made me ill. I felt fine interviewing Maryam and have no idea why I'm suddenly so unwell. The professor walks in and greets us with a warm smile, insisting we call him Sandy. I'm supposed to ask detailed questions about PTSD and the brain, but mine has stopped working. As Helen fixes a microphone to his tie, I ask Sandy what he thinks is happening to me.

'Going to Ward 17 takes you back to very specific memories and recollections about why you have PTSD and that must evoke many of those memories. There is a whole neuro-circuitry involved in memory that we know a great deal about,' Sandy says. 'The second thing is that Melbourne is a very busy place. One of the things we know about the brain and PTSD is that people can't order and structure information the same way they previously could. So being put in a high intensity environment really challenges your ability to filter information and if you can't filter information you become overwhelmed because there is just a world of noise and physical inputs that you can't manage.'

I'm not going crazy! This scholarly, down-to-earth man in his mid-60s makes me feel a bit better, enough to carry on.

Sandy says some changes to the brain from PTSD are irreversible and can be measured, even before people are diagnosed. In fact, a study of Australian troops deployed to the Middle East had shown this, he tells us. They had significant abnormalities in working memory, in their ability to structure and organise verbal information. Once someone had PTSD, additional changes could be documented that showed the brain couldn't work as an integrated unit.

'The brain is like a symphony orchestra. With PTSD, it's like the conductor has fallen off the podium,' Sandy adds.

'Sorry, you're saying these changes to the brain are permanent?' I ask, appalled.

'To a significant degree, yes,' he replies. 'I think first responders probably have more intense exposure than troops because they don't have periods of respite. There is a substantial body of evidence that shows first responders have a loss of total brain volume. So, it's not just about the way their structures are talking to each other.'

It's like your brain shrinks over time, Sandy says.

I literally can't believe what Sandy says about first responders because it's so shocking. I think of my mates in Ward 17. This is a bloody crisis.

Sandy then talks about research he'd done into survivors of the 1983 Ash Wednesday bushfires that killed 75 people in South Australia and Victoria. What most stood out was their trouble concentrating.

'That's not what people generally complain of. People complain of nightmares and horrific memories, so I got intrigued in what lay behind that difficulty in focusing on information,' he says.

Sandy had earlier told me that if he gave me a series of facts to organise and came back to me several minutes later, I wouldn't be able to use the information as well as someone without PTSD.

Some of my managers half-jokingly used to say I could do the work of two people because of my stamina and focus. Right now, in March 2017, a typical eight-hour day is a challenge. Completing tasks is vital to our self-worth, whatever our occupation. It's also necessary to keep our jobs.

The problem is the perception that PTSD equals damaged goods. Employers can't see inside our brains, but they know what we used to do, and they will try to guess what we're capable of now. All this affects keeping your job, getting back to work, or getting a new job.

It's time to finish the interview with Sandy.

One last question: 'Why is it that the public seems to know so little about the profound impact PTSD can have on first responders and soldiers?'

'One of the enormous difficulties someone like myself faces is the lack of the use of knowledge we have by people who should know about that information,' Sandy replies evenly. 'I am talking about emergency service administrators and DVA. We haven't fully embraced the knowledge we have. As a consequence, I think we are living with a 20th century understanding of this disorder in the face of 21st century knowledge. I think that is inexcusable.'

It is a damning indictment from a man who has tried for decades to get the Australian Defence Force, Department of Veterans' Affairs and first responder organisations to take better care of their people. DVA and the ADF, under the government of Prime Minister Scott Morrison, stopped funding the Centre for Traumatic Stress Studies at the end of 2019, forcing it to close.

Helen drops me at an Airbnb in the city where I take Panadol and sleep for a few hours. I set my alarm for 9.30 pm because she will film me interviewing Bessel van der Kolk at 11 pm.

It's taken a month of endless emails with his assistant in Boston for me to set this up.

I feel so sick, I want to cry. I cancel the interview.

I see Wendy a few days later. I've shelved the idea of going to Baghdad. If visiting Ward 17 and Melbourne triggered me so badly, how on earth could I travel to Iraq? It's my third session with Wendy. We haven't gotten close to trying Adaptive Disclosure. I can't talk about Namir and Saeed. I can barely open my mouth. Wendy says I'm struggling with therapy in the 'real world' outside Ward 17. Mary thinks I should return as a patient.

'Of course, this would be a disaster,' I tell Helen Barrow in an email.

I didn't think for a second I'd need to go back as a patient. While I'd connected with the veterans and coppers, many on repeat admissions, I thought I'd be different: my family was behind me, I had an amazing new role at Reuters, my life had renewed meaning. But it was more than that. A year ago, I couldn't comprehend having PTSD. Mental illness wasn't part of my identity. Having accepted the need for treatment, I threw 25 years of journalism at the problem. In Ward 17, I was Dean Yates the journo again, working twelve hours a day, asking questions, reading and writing. Getting to the bottom of my illness. Going back as a patient wouldn't be part of the new identity I was subconsciously forging. Arrogance played its part: I thought I was intelligent enough to need one admission only. Returning would mean failure. Not even a year had passed since my discharge.

Anyone who seeks in-patient treatment for psychiatric illness or addiction should be applauded. It's an act of strength.

—

Two months later in mid-June, ABC journalist Ginny Stein flies to Tasmania. Ginny, an old friend, is working for the *Lateline* program (which gets axed at the end of 2017) and wants to do a story on my journey. We drive to the rainforest, where Ginny manoeuvres a drone through canopy to get shots of me on a footbridge across a river. I feel sick as the day goes on. I know Ginny will ask about the tenth anniversary of Namir and Saeed's deaths, just a month away on 12 July. My anxiety spikes, though I don't say anything. In the end, I handle Ginny's questions reasonably well.

The next day I start going downhill. Headaches and neck pain that will last nearly three weeks. The slightest noise sets me off. I can't think straight. Exhaustion.

A few days later, Mary says she thinks I need to go back to Ward 17 to get through the anniversary. I reluctantly agree. My new role at Reuters was announced internally the previous month. *How the hell will that look?* My manager is the chief operating officer, but I also work closely with the global head of HR, both based in New York. They are very supportive and tell me to take as much time as I need. Reuters will pay for the admission. The contrast to how I was treated previously is uplifting. The company has my back. I can focus on myself.

The following day I only get through half a 90-minute indoor Bikram Yoga class. I lie down in 42-degree heat, the temperature setting for this form a yoga. What a failure.

As my second admission draws closer, the notion of my role in Namir and Saeed's deaths begins to form in my head. 'My role': words I start using for the first time. Then comes the word 'complicit'. I'm not sure where I'm going with this, but I know I'll need to bare my soul in Ward 17. Write that letter to Namir and Saeed, watch Collateral Murder, and unlock my emotions. The one that needs no key is anger.

Until I got PTSD I wouldn't have described myself as an angry person.

At Reuters, I was the correspondent, bureau chief and editor every manager seemed to want. Good news judgement, calm under pressure. When Reuters needed to reinforce Indonesia in 2000 during political chaos and violence, I was asked to relocate from Hanoi, where I was a young bureau chief. In late 2006, with civil war raging in Iraq, I was asked to apply for the job of running the Baghdad operation. At the time I'd been based in Jerusalem for only nine months as deputy bureau chief for Israel and Palestine. The bosses never doubted my leadership, even when Crazy Horse 1–8 killed Namir and Saeed. There was no internal inquiry. I had to conduct my own nearly a decade later. At one point, with violence off the charts in Baghdad in 2007, the then editor-in-chief said to me in an email: 'If at any time you feel we need to take drastic action like an evacuation [of the bureau]. Just whisper the word and it's done. You have my absolute 100% confidence in making the right decisions.' When Reuters created the job of top news editor in Asia in 2010, I was asked to fill that role.

PTSD and moral injury changed everything.

Anger is now my default, my 'safe' emotion. That is partly because PTSD has rewired my nervous system. Then there is my rage at Reuters, the betrayal, the moral injury. I suspect my anger is also linked to identity. The journalist whose passion for the job was widely admired by his bosses and colleagues is gone.

Who am I now?

14

Ritual, remembrance
and absolution

From the taxi, I see Ward 17 a short distance away, but it's dream-like. I was here three months ago with the filmmakers. Now I'm back as a patient. I shake my head in disbelief as I pull my suitcases behind me. It's 28 June 2017.

In my notebook on the flight to Melbourne, I wrote:

- *How do journalists heal from moral injury? Are there retreats?*
- *Purification/Cleansing.*
- *Letter/Namir and Saeed. Talk to them?*
- *How can I honour their memory so they won't be forgotten?*
- *What would they want me to do?*
- *Need to undertake a healing journey.*
- *Watch WikiLeaks tape. Need to feel emotion.*
- *Email Brett Litz, talk to Chelsea Manning.*
- *Where is this going to lead?*

I go through the motions of admission, unpack in Room 15. I feel unwell all afternoon, fragile and vulnerable. My blood pressure is high. That night Mary puts me on speaker so I can talk to her and the kids. Belle had the wood-fired heater going when Mary got home from work.

I sleep poorly. My three-week-old headache hasn't budged.

Dr Maryam is on twelve months maternity leave. While I'm thrilled for Maryam, her absence worries me. I'm sure I could write my letter under her care and guidance. An older psychiatrist filling in sees me the next morning. His jolly personality puts me off. Worse, he's never heard of moral injury. I keep the session short and ask for another psychiatrist. I then see an in-house psychologist in her early 30s who I'll call Natalie. She wasn't here during my first admission. I like Natalie, who wants to help patients find meaning from their trauma.

She knows some of my history. I say that when I wept after Namir and Saeed were killed, it was because my Iraqi colleagues thought less of me. I don't think it was grief. It was about me. How selfish. Natalie says my emotions are intellectualised, buried deep. She thinks my standards are unrelenting as opposed to high.

Yes, I've heard that before, I reply.

I tell her about my list, the people I want to contact.

'Don't do anything yet,' Natalie advises. 'Get your nervous system under control. Walk. Do yoga. Drop the urgency. You could collapse.'

'Can I do some Reuters work?'

'What? No! This must be about you. How can you encourage your colleagues to practise self-care if you don't?'

To my dismay, Natalie says she will be on leave next week. Today is Thursday. Use the time for self-care, she urges. I consider flying home and coming back when she returns. Then I think, okay, I'll exercise, read, build playlists on Spotify, and watch rugby league matches. Try to work through this stuff myself.

Social worker Christina Sim comes to see me late that afternoon.

'We knew you'd be back,' she says. 'Last year you were still numb. You were in crisis. We wanted you to slow down. Being here sends a positive message that it's okay to have a relapse.'

She laughs when I tell her about wanting to work. Natalie had already told her.

'You're on a journey,' Christina says. 'You're trying to do so much when you're still recovering.'

I feel a bit better.

I talk to Michelle, the OT. Get back into your routine, she says.

As usual, Ward 17 is quiet the following day, Friday. I'm reading *War and the Soul: Healing Our Nation's Veterans From Post-Traumatic Stress Disorder* by American clinical psychotherapist Edward Tick, for a second time. Tick is on my list of people to email. In his book, published in 2005, Tick writes that US veterans have been through a profound death-rebirth process and are significantly and permanently transformed. Extreme damage has been done to their character. As such, PTSD should be seen as an identity disorder and soul wound, affecting personality at the deepest level.

Western societies expect veterans to put war behind them and become ordinary citizens again, writes Tick. It's impossible. Veterans live in a 'frozen war consciousness'. This is what Vietnam veteran and fellow Ward 17 patient Ray Watson meant when he told me he couldn't stop living in 1966.

Veterans are given little opportunity to rebuild dignity and rediscover inner peace, says Tick. In contrast to traditional cultures, modern treatments exclude sacred and communal dimensions of healing. And the recovery of an individual isn't a priority because the system functions despite the loss of significant numbers of the adult population. That's one reason why no one has been held accountable in Australia for the countless suicides among veterans and first responders, for the thousands more who are mentally scarred: young recruits will always be eager to fill their shoes.

'Post-traumatic stress disorder is our modern metaphor for the condition of soul sickness; the quasi-scientific name allows us to find a place for it among the psychological categories we use today to analyze the human experience,' Tick writes.

Identity transformation is one of the deeper dimensions of PTSD, adds Tick. Identity wound is probably a more apt description, I think. It's something I've been grappling with since my PTSD diagnosis, since going on sick leave, believing my journalism career was finished. But it goes back further.

My life had immense purpose until we moved to Evandale in early 2013. After that, all I did was edit stories in my study. Run the odd news-planning call. I had little face-to-face contact with people outside my family except when I took my kids to school and sport. I needed a broader mission, where I was proud of what I was doing.

My identity began to disintegrate after I went on sick leave in early 2016. As stressful as my editing job had become, it gave my life structure. I was highly respected by colleagues, who often sought my advice. Then I dropped off the radar for seven months. Before long, I knew I couldn't return to journalism. It was a combination of feeling incapable of doing the work and finding it meaningless.

It will take years to fully understand the significance of my identity wound. But it makes sense this should be front and centre of trauma therapy. How can treatment work if you don't know who you are?

For years, Tick has taken veterans to Vietnam to facilitate ceremonies, rituals and meetings with former North Vietnamese soldiers to open the way for forgiveness and understanding. Recovery requires purification, storytelling, healing journeys and grieving rituals. One of the most powerful practices is the Native American sweat lodge, a centuries-old tradition, Tick says. Its purposes included purification of warriors on their return from battle.

I put Tick's book down on the bed and recall my British friend Matthew Green had written a magazine article about going to sweat lodges. Matt and I have been exchanging emails and chatting on Skype since Reuters published my special report in November, but we haven't been in touch for a couple of months. I google sweat lodges in Melbourne. Freakishly, there is one a few suburbs from Ward 17 that holds weekly sweats. The experience is about birth, death, rebirth and creating a new internal balance. The sweat fosters peace, self-worth and can help with trauma. That grabs my attention. I call the organiser and sign up for Monday evening.

I write Matt a brief email, saying I'm back in Ward 17 and planning a sweat as part of ways to heal over Namir and Saeed, including 'my role' in their deaths. Younger than me by seven years, Matt lives in London. He has covered war in Iraq, Afghanistan and Africa. He also wrote about less mainstream methods to treat trauma in his brilliant 2015 book on British veterans, *Aftershock: The Untold Story of Surviving Peace*.

Matt replies quickly, saying he normally wouldn't give unsolicited advice, but will risk it with me.

'Create a strong intention about what you want to let go of in the lodge (guilt, anger, sadness). Also, what you want to "'bring in'" (peace, clarity, courage). Perhaps there is something you need to say to Namir and Saeed. Maybe you need to listen for what they have to say to you.'

Matt doesn't directly address 'my role' in his reply, so I spell it out. It's the first time I've done this for anyone, including myself, in written form:

'It's not that I want to let go of the guilt,' I write. 'I want to say I'm sorry that I never asked the US military for its rules of engagement. Had I done that, Namir and Saeed would be alive. I would have been able to tell my staff that hanging around armed men would risk getting shot and killed. I also want to honour Namir and Saeed. I'm thinking of writing a Facebook blog for 12 July that will pay homage to them, and other journalists who've been killed that I knew. I want to ask Namir and Saeed for forgiveness. I want to ask them how they want me to lead my life.'

Matt doesn't think I need to dive into the details, the story of what happened in Baghdad, during my sweat. I could keep it as simple as creating a strong intention to do what is necessary to heal. That way, I set aside the thought process in the rational mind and create space for my unconscious to do its work. He likes the idea of a social media commemoration but invites me to consider a private ceremony of remembrance.

'And I love your last question. The sweat lodge would be a great place to ask for guidance from Namir and Saeed because it will help open up the more intuitive, even mystical side of the brain,' he says.

Matt has got me thinking. I wonder if I could also do something in the Heidelberg Repatriation Hospital chapel on 12 July. I leave a note at the nurses' station, asking to meet the Ward 17 chaplain.

That night I see an ABC story online that says American philosopher Nancy Sherman is visiting Australia. Nancy wrote a book called *Afterwar: Healing the Moral Wounds of Our Soldiers* and had also been on my list of people to contact. I've brought *Afterwar* with me. Like *War and the Soul*, I plan to read it again. One short sentence resonated with me before: moral wounds demand moral healing. I find Nancy's email address and send her a message. She agrees to chat the following morning.

Nancy calls *Afterwar* an intimate look at a handful of the 2.6 million American men and women who served in Iraq and Afghanistan. She writes about Corporal Eduardo 'Lalo' Panyagua, a marine veteran of Iraq, who blamed himself for the deaths of two marines killed by IEDs in Afghanistan. Panyagua was, as he put it, in charge of the combat area. Nancy writes that most people would say Panyagua's guilt was irrational and inappropriate. He was naive about what he could control or gripped by wishful thinking. But those veterans can only move forward in life once their guilt is recognised for what it is, with its 'moral pulls and aspirations, and its blurred vision'.

Nancy states: 'To call it irrational or recalcitrant can be dismissive, encouraging us to overlook the genuine figuring out that is often part of the psychological process of healthy ownership of moral responsibility. That process may include an investigative sorting out of the facts of the matter: a psychological working through of the conflicts, investments, losses; an acceptance of the limits of control that often are part of this kind of reflection.'

Thank you! Nancy had just validated what I've been doing at times over the past year, forensically assessing my actions and omissions.

Nancy and I speak for an hour. She is familiar with Collateral Murder and friends with several journalists who've experienced moral wounds from their reporting. I tell Nancy about the two worlds I inhabit.

'In one, there is disbelief I feel this way, ten years on. In the other, it overwhelms me. No one understands me,' I say.

We talk about anniversaries. These are difficult, retraumatising events, she says.

'What if you knew the ROEs and yet something happened, would you still feel responsible?' Nancy asks.

Not necessarily. I give the example of translator Lu'oy al-Joubouri, killed by militants. I never felt guilt over what happened to him. That was outside my control.

'You clearly feel you need to atone,' she adds.

I'm supposed to go to the sweat lodge that evening, but I postpone. The timing isn't right. My brain is too busy.

———

The following day, I buy an A4 notepad and begin handwriting my letter to Namir and Saeed. I'd planned to type it on my laptop, but a friend suggested doing it by hand.

Dear Namir & Saeed – I have wanted to write this letter for a long time . . .

A nurse knocks on my door to say the chaplain has arrived. I walk into the common room and see an attractive woman with streaks of white through her shoulder-length hair at the nurses' station. She is wearing bright coloured clothes and red lipstick. *That can't be the chaplain.* I walk over and say hello. Her name is Cath Taylor, the Ward 17 spiritual care worker. Cath tells me she is doing final chaplaincy studies. She is 32 and used to be a fashion designer but switched careers because she felt unfulfilled.

We go to the small TV room where I watch rugby league

on weekends alone – Ward 17 is the domain of Australian rules football. Cath knows nothing about me, so I give her a summary. She sees guilt and shame often; she understands moral injury. Not enough attention is paid to the possible spiritual journey out of trauma, she says. To persuade Vietnam veterans to do mindfulness meditation, she tells them: 'The army taught you how to go to war. I'm going to teach you how to live.'

Cath and I talk about holding a ceremony at the chapel on 12 July for Namir and Saeed. She suggests I use the occasion to pay my respects. We could light candles, she says. I could buy my own. I tell Cath I'd like to read aloud the letter I'm writing. I'll also get photos of Namir and Saeed printed. Cath calls what we are planning a ritual. I see it as a memorial service.

I also look for answers in Islam, the religion practised by Namir and Saeed. The Elsedeaq Heidelberg Mosque is 2–3 kilometres from Ward 17. *The Age* newspaper ran a nice profile on its young, two-metre tall imam earlier this year. Alaa El Zokm lives opposite the mosque. That afternoon, I walk to his modest brick home. He answers after a couple of knocks.

I introduce myself in faltering Arabic, saying I'm a journalist. The Egyptian-born cleric is unfazed by this stranger talking about two Iraqi men killed in Baghdad a decade earlier. He knows Collateral Murder and invites me in. At 28, he seems young for an imam. But I sense wisdom underneath the youthful demeanour.

Alaa sits opposite me and serves tea.

'How can I help?' he asks.

I tell him my story then ask if he can forgive people. Only Allah can forgive, not an imam, he replies, before insisting the deaths of Namir and Saeed were not my fault. He's not interested in the details. It was their destiny. God's will. Their deaths were pre-ordained. The word 'pre-ordained' reminds me of what I'd often heard in the Muslim world. That events, especially tragic ones, were the will of Allah.

That won't work for me, I need something concrete.

'So, what can I do?' I say.

Alaa talks about the five pillars of Islam – faith, prayer, charity, fasting and the pilgrimage to Mecca. As I'm a non-Muslim, Alaa suggests charity, or *zakat*. I can donate on behalf of Namir and Saeed.

'Should this be to the Muslim community?' I ask.

Alaa laughs, saying it can be to anyone or any organisation. 'If I need a blood transfusion, I'm not going to ask for Muslim blood!'

I smile at his humour then ask if I can attend Friday prayers. I want to reconnect with Muslim people and culture.

'You are welcome,' he replies, opening his massive arms.

I thank Alaa for his advice. On the way back to Ward 17, he sends me a friend request on Facebook which I immediately accept.

It's been a good day. I have much writing to do. And I have the ceremony on 12 July. I can devote time, energy and, hopefully, emotion to that. And I'm gaining insight into my moral injury.

I have another wonderful talk with Cath. I ask if she has symbols of Islam she can bring to the chapel. While I'm not religious, I want to link Christianity with Islam in the service. Mary has suggested I find a prayer from the Koran. Cath says the ritual could be a way to release ten years of accumulated guilt and shame.

'While I know it's not the right word to use, I feel excited,' I say.

'It's your anticipation of doing something very meaningful for Namir and Saeed,' she replies.

Just before I leave Ward 17 and walk to the mosque for midday prayers on Friday, Mary emails me some notes and a quote from the Koran, which she has used when counselling Muslim clients: Allah decides the appointed time when someone passes from this life to the next, the Koran emphasises. In grief there must be patience (*sabr*) and acceptance, Mary writes. This might help my healing. In commemorating Namir and Saeed's deaths, I could ask for '*sabr*', Mary says. It's perfect.

The mosque is a nondescript building, the size of a large home. Most of the faithful are from Somalia, as well as parts of the Middle East and the Asian sub-continent. I feel self-conscious and decide not to go inside. A man is laying mats across the courtyard, so I figure men will pray there as well. I'm fifteen minutes early. Young boys stare at me, but not the men.

Soon the courtyard is packed. Latecomers, taxi drivers, park their vehicles and remove their shoes then wash their feet, hands and faces under communal taps. Alaa arrives wearing robes.

It's been a long time since I've heard the call to prayer. I sit among the worshippers. Alaa delivers his sermon in a mix of English and Arabic. My mind roams the many years I spent in the Muslim world. I notice a man sitting a few rows in front of me. From behind, he looks like Saeed.

That afternoon I pick up framed photos of Namir and Saeed from a shop in Ivanhoe. One shows images of them on a large screen outside the Thomson Reuters building in London. The owner, curious, politely asks what the photos are for. After I explain, he says: 'I hope Ward 17 does what it can for you. I hope I too have done my bit in a small way.'

I thank him for his kindness.

On Sunday, I prepare for the sweat lodge. I'm nervous and excited. I get a taxi to the venue in East Brunswick. The lodge is four-foot high, built on sand. About a dozen men and women crawl in anti-clockwise. I'm wearing just a sarong. It's cramped, not enough room to sit cross-legged around the heated stones. Peter, the lodge leader, pours water on the rocks which creates steam and more heat. I want to give my guilt and shame to the heat, as well as the grip the events of 12 July 2007 have on me. I want self-forgiveness from the stones.

Peter talks about spiritual journeys. We chant. While I like the ritual, the heat is intense. My heart races. My throat burns. My hair, when I touch it, feels like it's on fire, and this is just the first of three sessions.

Halfway through the second session I'm done. Peter is on my right. I have to leave, I whisper, crawling out. I'm so dizzy I hunch over on the sand for a minute before standing up. The ground sways. I suck in cold winter air, drink water and lie on a bench in the evening darkness.

Back at Ward 17, drained, I go to bed.

The next morning Cath and I have a final catch-up before the memorial service in two days. She has put much thought into it. One loose end for me is eight little handmade wooden blue wrens that Mary sent the week before. We often see blue wrens outside our living room windows in Evandale. I'd wanted a wren for Namir, Saeed and Lu'oy to represent their souls at the service. I don't need that many, I thought when I opened the box.

But as the days passed, I realised another four could represent the souls of Reuters journalists I worked with and who were also violently taken from this world: Australian cameraman Harry Burton, killed in Afghanistan; Iraqi cameraman Yasser Faisal, killed in Syria; and Iraqi journalists Muhanad Mohammed and Sabah al-Bazi, both killed in Iraq.

That leaves one wren, which has sat apart from the others on my windowsill for days. Then I realise it can represent my soul. Mary has always wanted me to see things more spiritually. 'You're a casualty of what happened in Baghdad too,' she says.

I finish my letter to Namir and Saeed. It's taken six days to write 4885 words. A bit over 22 pages.

I can't sleep that night and have a headache, so I go to the nurses' station to get some meds around 11.30 pm. A retired senior detective called Jo Donovan had come in a few days earlier. I spot Jo pacing the corridors, amped up. It's her first admission. I reassure Jo – who had been a copper for 27 years – saying it's normal to feel this way. Going back to my room, I absent-mindedly count the number of nights I've spent in Ward 17 in the past year: 49. No wonder I'm not doing the same.

I still have the headache when I get up the next morning, the eve of the anniversary. I'm tense. The anticipation about the service is gone, replaced by uneasiness. Maybe it's the unknown.

'What's the worst thing that can happen?' a nurse asks.

'That I get emotional and cry,' I say, immediately correcting myself, since that's *exactly* what I want. No, the worst thing will be not feeling anything. That would tell me this was all about me and not Namir and Saeed. That I was mourning the bureau chief I thought I was.

*

On the day of the ceremony, I wake around 6 am and go for a long walk to clear my head. At breakfast, anxiety spreads across my chest. Luckily, Helen Barrow arrives after a red-eye flight from Sydney. I want Helen to film so people understand how I'm trying to heal from my moral injury. When it's time to go, I place the two framed photographs of Namir and Saeed in a small box along with candles and the eight blue wrens. Cath is waiting outside the Anzac Memorial Chapel on the ground floor of one of the hospital wings. The chapel's windows are stained glass. Plaques and flags representing Australian military campaigns adorn the walls. It's a peaceful place. Because Helen is filming on hospital grounds, a member of the PR team from Austin Health, which runs the hospital, is there. Helen mics me up, asking what I hope to get from the service. The PR flak sits so close that Helen asks her to move. The woman says she needs to hear my answers, as if I might badmouth Ward 17 in the chapel. When Helen films Cath and me setting up, she keeps getting in the frame. Helen hisses at her. The flak tells Cath to pin her Austin Health name badge to her shirt, so it's visible. Remarkably, I don't lose my cool.

I put the photos of Namir and Saeed on the altar together with three small candles and three blue wrens. The remaining five wrens go to one side. Cath places a large candle on the altar for me and some tapers. She lays a Muslim prayer mat on the floor and uses her iPhone to find the direction of Mecca, Islam's holiest city.

We're ready. Cath stands next to me, the order of service on her iPad. She reads a blessing by Irishman John O'Donohue, a poet and philosopher, then asks me to begin. I take a deep breath.

(Excerpts)

Dear Namir and Saeed,

I need to get straight to the point, my friends.

I believe that if I'd been a better bureau chief you would both be alive today. My most important role was staff safety. The story was second.

I cannot understand why I didn't ask the US military for a copy of its rules of engagement. Okay, they may not have given me one, but I'm sure they would have briefed me on the key points so that I could keep you both and all the other staff as safe as possible.

It could have been as simple as that. I should have just asked: what are the key things I need to know to protect my staff? I never did that, and I believe it cost you both your lives.

None of my predecessors talked about the ROEs from memory. Nor did any of the chief editors in London. That should not have made any difference. We were operating in the world's most dangerous country. Scores of journalists had been killed already. I'd arrived in Baghdad six months earlier, so it wasn't like I was new. I'd arrived a few weeks before the so-called surge of US troops got underway. That first six months of 2007 was the bloodiest period of the war. The US military was really going after al-Qaeda in Iraq and other insurgents.

I knew all this and yet I still didn't ask the US military for a briefing on how the ROEs could affect my staff.

About ten days ago, a thought occurred to me: If Reuters had held an inquiry into your deaths, the person leading it would have asked: 'The US military said its ROEs allowed soldiers to open fire on armed men in the streets of Baghdad. Did the bureau chief ever ask the military for an understanding of its ROEs?' The answer would have been no. A gross dereliction of duty? Perhaps. Contributing to the tragic deaths of both of you? A reasonable answer would be YES.

You both might be wondering why it's taken me so long to get to a clear-headed understanding of this.

On August 15, 2016, I wrote a note for Dr Maryam, my psychiatrist during my first admission to Ward 17. She had asked me to explain in detail why I felt such guilt and shame over your deaths.

I mentioned the briefing with the generals in Baghdad. I wrote: 'Pilot mistakes Namir's camera for an RPG and opens fire. Video stops. I put my head in my hands . . . Irrespective of what Namir did to cast suspicion on himself, did the US military have the right to open fire? My reaction at the time was basically yes. Is this wrong? It sure feels wrong now. Should I have said this to the Iraqi staff? I feel guilt for even thinking that Namir's actions might have caused that tragic loss of life.'

Namir – I just cannot understand why I was thinking like this. They were going to attack whether you peered around that corner or not. The order had already been given. For me, nine years later, and at the time, to have blamed you is beyond comprehension.

I have done you, your good name and your family an enormous disservice to even suggest you were to blame.

I can't wind the clock back ten years. But I believe you would both want me to find meaning in my life. Words will never express how sorry I am that I failed to be a better bureau chief. That I failed to protect you both and that as a result you were both killed.

Namir and Saeed – I beg your forgiveness.

There are other things I feel guilt and shame about.

– After you were both killed, Mariam Karouny told me the Iraqi staff were upset because they felt I was soft on the military in our stories. I broke down and cried. But I was crying for me! I was not crying for you both. Why could I not show and feel the emotion I should have? My treating team here say I was numb. I know that's true, but it feels like a lame excuse.

– I did not mark the anniversary of your deaths until last year. Why? I suspect it was a defence mechanism, my avoidance. Still, it seems inconceivable that I could be so uncaring, so heartless, to have not even paused and remembered the two of you. Shame on me.

– Finally, when WikiLeaks released the tape in 2010, my response was pathetic. I think I was shocked. I felt duped by the two generals. I knew then why they had never given us the video. I could have made clear that permission to open fire had been given before you peered around the corner, Namir – thus avoiding the impression given by many in the media that it was the Apache mistaking your camera for an RPG that caused them to open fire. This annoyed Julian Assange, who later criticised the media for missing this vital point. Again, because of this, no questions were raised – NONE – about my conduct and whether I'd done everything to protect my staff.

It's time I finished, Namir and Saeed. I want to end with a quote from the Koran.

'Whatever we are given is a gift from Allah. We are not its owner. Everything belongs to Allah and returns to Him.'

I'd thought about reading this letter for days. I wanted to sob. As I read, I grew frustrated. Why am I not crying? What's wrong with me? My eyes were moist but not a drop rolled down my cheek. Was I too focused on the letter? Was it Helen and the camera?

Cath and I light the candles and tapers and step back. Cath catches me off-guard: do you want to say anything to Namir and Saeed? I step forward, look at their photo and ask them to forgive me. Cath reads a verse from scripture.

'If we freely confess our sins, God, the loving divine, faithful and just – rich in mercy – will forgive us our sins and cleanse us continually from all unrighteousness and wrongdoing.'

Cath asks me to place my hands over an empty stone bowl. I close my eyes. She slowly pours a jug of cold water over my hands. Suddenly, I'm in the Tarkine rainforest, my hands in the icy waters of a tannin-stained river. My mind is still. I'm cleansed.

Cath dips her index finger into oil and makes the sign of the cross on my forehead several times. Then she asks me to blow out the candles and tapers. Smoke from the large candle rises into the air. The disappearing smoke is my guilt and shame.

I sit on the windowsill in the chapel. I've honoured Namir and Saeed. A weight has lifted. I think I struggled between wanting to show emotion and making sure the hour-long service went smoothly, I tell Cath and Helen. 'Maybe you just need to let the emotion happen,' says Helen. Cath agrees. Cath says I'm a different person to the one she met ten days ago. She gives me a small copy of the Koran and Muslim prayer beads. I ask Cath if I can give her a hug. Of course, she says. The PR woman jumps in, saying Austin staff can't touch patients. Helen is filming. Seriously! Helen and I shake our heads in bemusement. I think Cath tries to keep a straight face. Helen turns the camera off and I hug Cath anyway.

I've had another remarkable journey in Ward 17. An idea for a simple service in the chapel became something far deeper. I think it's the work I did over the past two weeks that has healed me. The reflecting, writing the letter, talking to so many different people, going to the mosque, trying the sweat lodge. Maybe that was why I didn't break down – I'd subconsciously forgiven myself along the way. The ceremony with Cath sealed it. Cath will tell me later she planned the service so this would happen. I focused on Namir and Saeed. She focused on me.

I leave the chapel and walk into winter sunshine. I want to go home to my family, get on with life.

That night I sleep badly, waking nearly ten times. The next morning, I still want to fly home, but Mary urges me to stay several more days. After putting up a bit of a fight, I agree.

'Your mind might be ready but maybe your body is not,' Mary says. 'Rest, reflect and write.'

I briefly leave the ward for some reason. When I get back, Cath has slipped the order of service under my door. It's an A4 page folded in half. On the front are two blue wrens facing each other; 12 July Two Thousand Seventeen are written underneath in capital letters. On the inside page are the words Ritual, Remembrance and Absolution. The text is a mix of blue and black, the colour of my little winged friends. On the back page is the blessing. I'm so touched. I stand the order of service on the windowsill next to the photos of Namir and Saeed, the wrens and the prayer beads.

I don't dwell on Namir and Saeed that day, the next nor the day after. My mind is clear.

Journal entry. Ward 17, Melbourne. July 14, 2017: My culpability only became crystal clear in Ward 17. Is that why I now feel so much better? I got to the root of it? I don't feel the need to go to Baghdad, watch the WikiLeaks tape.

I write an email to family and friends about the service. Cait McMahon from the Dart Center says emotions don't have to be expressed in tears.

'I am only realising this now,' I reply. 'I put so much pressure on myself ahead of the ceremony to display emotion that it distracted me until we got to the end. The last few days have been amazing. I shake my head as I write this, but I feel healed. Still much to reflect on and integrate of course.'

I type up my letter to Namir and Saeed to send to Mary. On two occasions, I type 'I felt guilt', instead of 'I feel guilt' as I wrote in the letter. My guilt is past tense in my subconscious. When Mary reads the email, she replies: 'I can now say, for the first time, that I truly understand your moral injury.'

I meet Cath the morning before I fly home. We can't stop smiling.

'Do you believe I've forgiven myself?'

'What do you think?'

'Yes.'

'Your journey here is complete.'

—

Unlike my first discharge when I struggled immediately, my second homecoming is smooth. I'm unburdened. No headaches or anxiety. I sleep well and return to work after a few days. I put a short post on Facebook about my experience. But some people respond saying the deaths of Namir and Saeed were not my fault. It was war.

It's easy to identify with someone's grief, anger or joy. Most people talk openly about such emotions. Less so with guilt, and harder still with shame. People feel very uncomfortable around shame. It's easier to tell people what we think they want to hear. No one wants to make a vulnerable person feel bad about themselves.

I decide to write another special report for Reuters, hoping that will help. I headline it: *Making Peace with the Dead: How a Chaplain and an Imam Healed My Soul.* I don't pitch the story.

I just write it and send it to Mike Williams and Alix Freedman in New York, saying I won't mind if it's not good enough, or the first-person narrative novelty has worn off. Mike gives the story the go-ahead as a follow-up special report.

I send a draft to a few Reuters colleagues for feedback. One is Andy Cawthorne, at the time running the Andean region, which includes the mess that is Venezuela. Andy is my age and has been based in Caracas for eight years. He's spent his career on the road in Africa and Latin America, seen a lot of death and misery. He replies that he was really struck by this sentence: 'Therein lies a key problem for people with moral injury. Everyone wants to make you feel better. It prolongs the pain.'

Obviously, so true, says Andy. That's one reason I want to get the story out there, I say. Everyone wants to be supportive, but for me it's been isolating.

Writing the new special report throws up a dilemma. I want to get the chronology of the deaths of Namir and Saeed correct to the second. In the first one I kept the description general to avoid watching Collateral Murder. I briefly consider asking a colleague to help, then decide it's my story. My job.

It takes a few seconds to find the footage on the internet. I minimise the video and mute the volume. It's October 2017, more than ten years since the two American generals showed me the first few minutes of the tape in Baghdad. Six months since Dr Maryam told me that was the most traumatising thing to happen in my career. I'd never reflected on it like that before. I'd focused on the day Namir and Saeed were killed. But Maryam was right. Nothing tortured me more than those few minutes in Saddam's former Republican Palace.

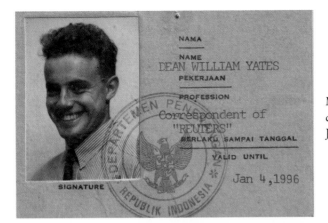

My Indonesian press
card. I joined Reuters in
Jakarta in late 1993.

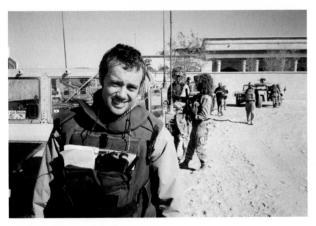

Left and below:
Embedded with US
troops searching for
Saddam Hussein near
Tikrit in late 2003.

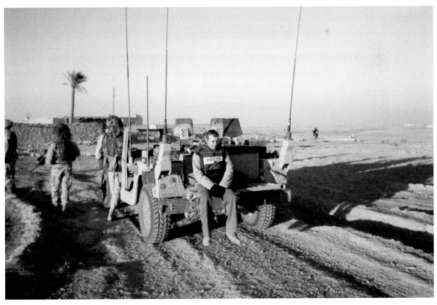

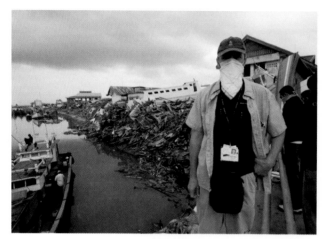

Left: The 2004 Boxing Day tsunami was beyond comprehension – 166,000 people killed in 20 minutes. Here, in the aftermath, people stare down at bodies tangled in debris in a Banda Aceh canal.

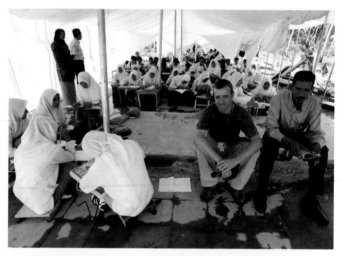

Right: Visiting a makeshift classroom a few weeks after the tsunami.

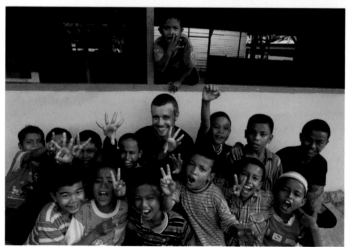

Joking around with boys at a camp for displaced people in Banda Aceh.

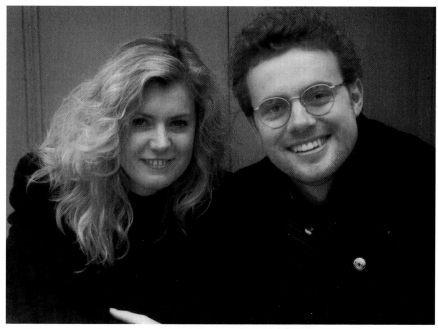

I met Mary in Hong Kong in 1995. We loved travelling together. This photo was taken in Macau in 1996.

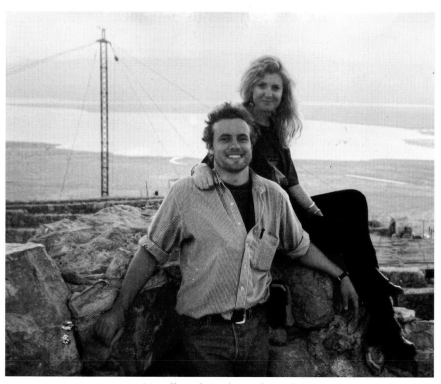

Travelling through Israel, 1996.

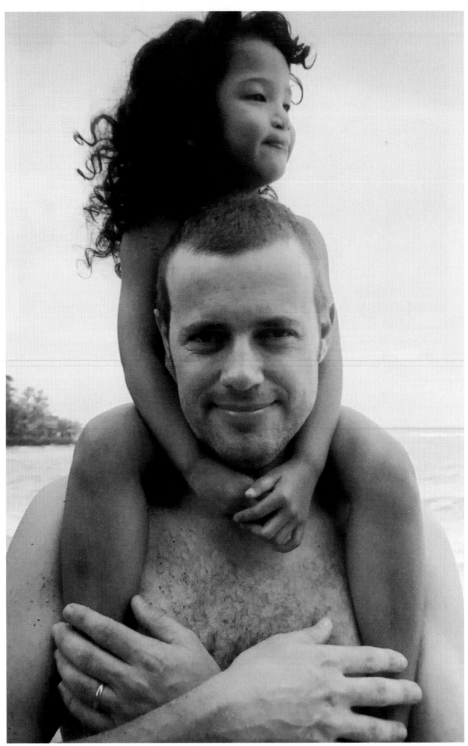

Belle and I at a beach in West Java, 2004.

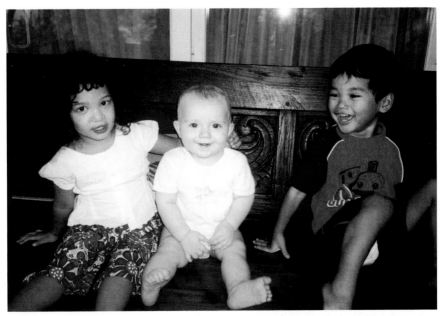

While I often travelled when the kids were young, I loved being with them. They brought me such joy. Belle, Harry and Patrick at home in Jakarta, 2003.

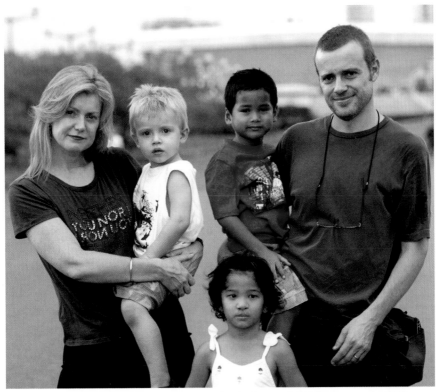

Family photo taken near the Reuters office before we left Jakarta in early 2006.

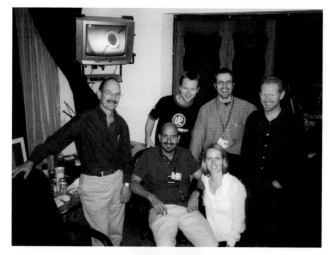

Left: On my first Baghdad assignment in late 2003, I was more concerned about doing a good job than getting killed. A boyish looking Andrew Marshall is on my right.

Right: I interviewed General David Petraeus, the then US military commander for Iraq, on several occasions, but never asked him about Namir and Saeed's deaths.

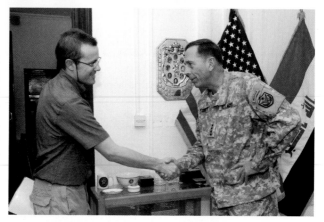

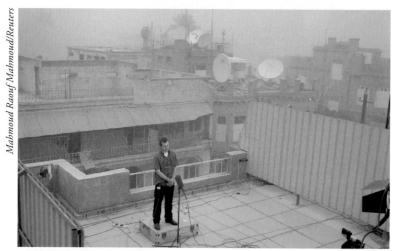

Preparing for a live broadcast on the roof of the Reuters bureau in Baghdad during a duststorm, 2008.

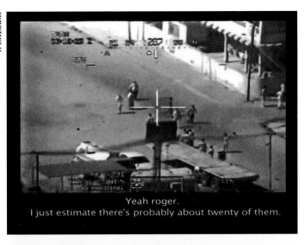

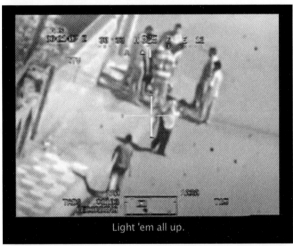

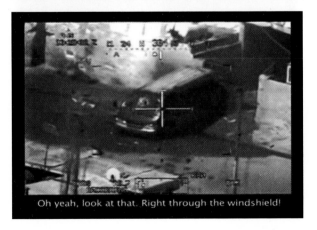

Collateral Murder footage – a sequence of events.

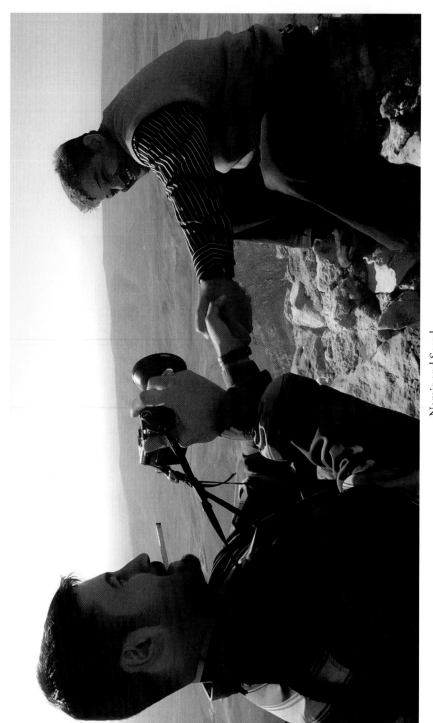

Namir and Saeed.

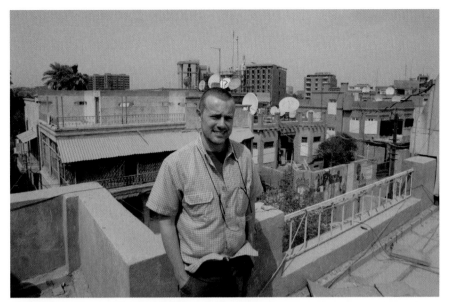

I had mixed emotions leaving Baghdad. I'd told Mary no more dangerous assignments. Pictured here on the roof of the Reuters house, 2008.

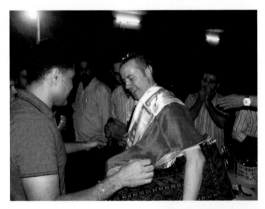

Left: The bureau threw me a touching farewell party. I told the Iraqi staff I'd look back on my posting as the most rewarding of my career. Staff gave me an Iraqi national flag they had all signed.

Right: Standing with some of the staff in the bureau yard. Mariam Karouny, my young deputy, is pictured left.

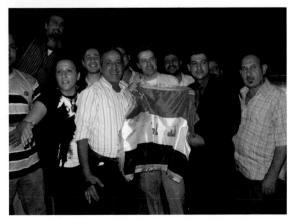

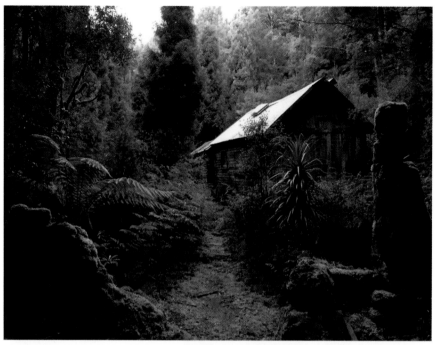

The Tarkine rainforest in Tasmania was where I found peace from the war in my head and chaos at home. Fraser Creek Hut was like a scene from *The Hobbit*.

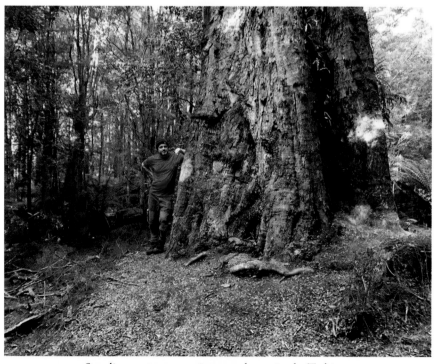

Standing next to an ancient myrtle tree in the Tarkine.

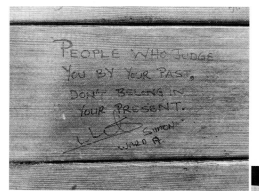

Left: Going to Ward 17 was a turning point in my life, but I worried whether the veterans and other patients would welcome a journalist. Then I noticed the messages scratched on the old coffee table.

Right: My room in Ward 17 on my first admission. A lot of hardwork got done in there.

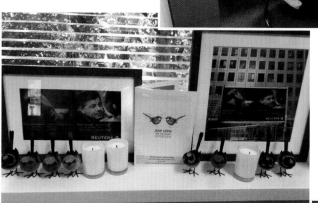

Left: Some of the items I placed on the altar for my memorial ceremony for Namir and Saeed during my second admission to Ward 17.

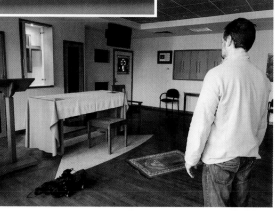

Right: Getting ready for the ceremony for Namir and Saeed in the Anzac Memorial Chapel.

Helen Barrow

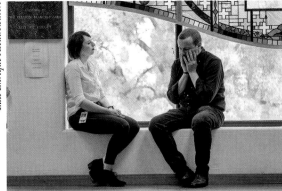

Left: Reflecting with Ward 17 spiritual care worker Cath Taylor a year after making peace with Namir and Saeed.

Luis Enrique Ascui/Reuters

Right: Chatting with imam Alaa El Zokm inside the Elsedeaq Heidelberg Mosque about the guidance he'd given me the previous year.

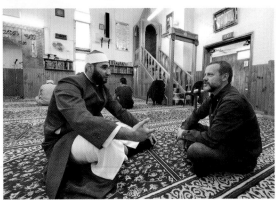

Luis Enrique Ascui/Reuters

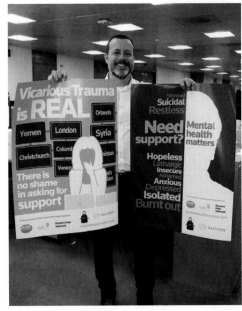

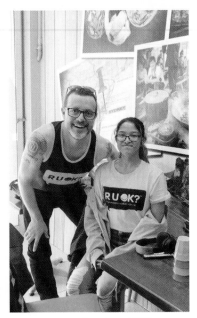

Above left: Advocating for mental health in the Reuters newsroom, London, 2019.
Above right: With Belle after giving a talk in Sydney to mark 'R U OK?' Day, 2019.

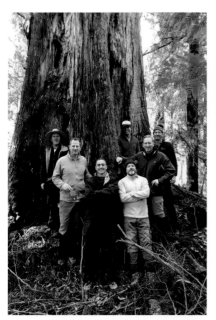

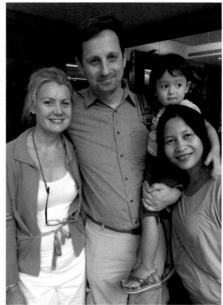

Top left: PTSD made me isolate myself. After I wrote my first story for Reuters about my struggles my old uni mates came to see me. Some I hadn't seen in 20 years. Every year we meet up to go bushwalking, often in the Tarkine.

Our friends Jeremy, Sari and Tessa have been incredibly supportive. They were a real rock for Mary. *Top right:* Jeremy, Sari and their daughter Charlotte pictured here with Mary, 2013.

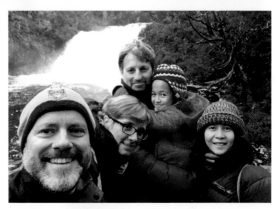

Middle right: At the Cradle Mountain National Park in 2018 with Jeremy, Sari, Charlotte and Tessa.

Bottom right: Sari, Tessa and Mary having fun on a Tassie holiday in 2016.

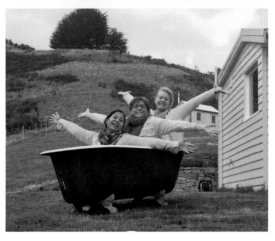

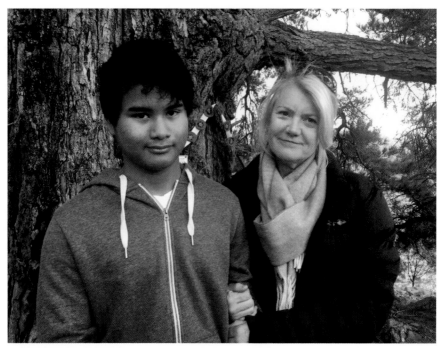

Patrick and Mary, 2016.

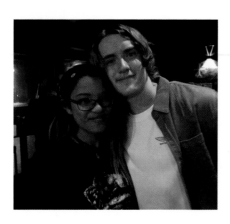

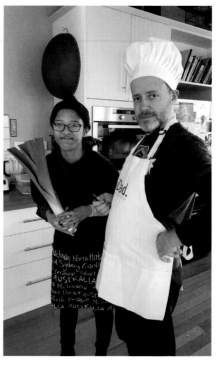

Above: Belle and Harry after Harry's band, Frogs in Suits, played their first pub gig in Hobart, 2021.

Right: Playing the clown in the kitchen, with Belle at home in Evandale, 2019.

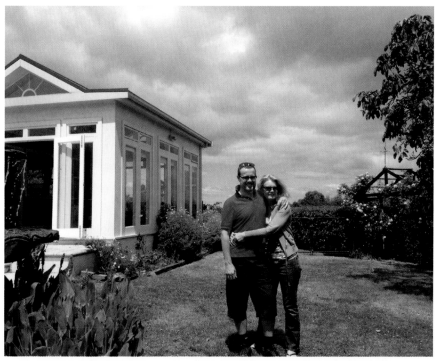

Mary and I soon after moving into our home in Evandale in early 2013.

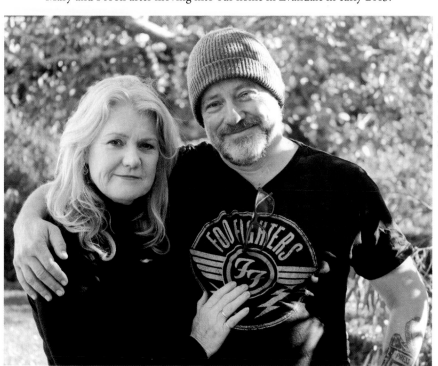

And ten years later, home, April 2023.

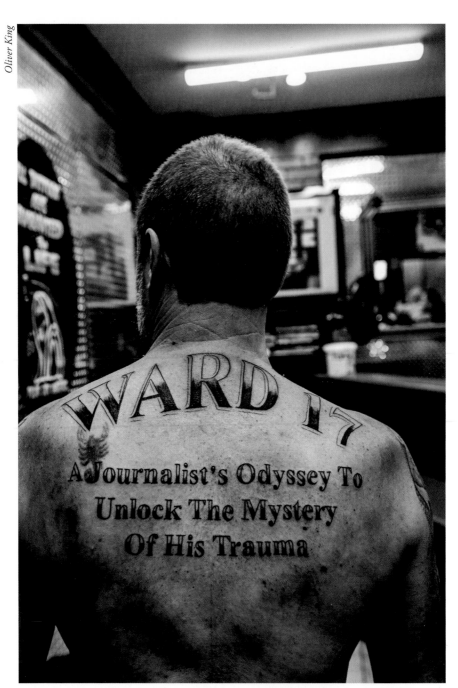

I promised myself a significant tattoo when I got a publishing deal. This was my proposed book title. It didn't work as a negotiating tactic . . .

I watch Namir look around the corner, barrage after barrage from Crazy Horse 1–8 smashing into men, Saeed struggling to get up. I know I've got my journalist's hat on, but I'm disconnected from what's happening on the screen.

Everything changes when I unmute the volume.

Gunner: 'Hotel 2–6, Crazy Horse 1–8. Have five to six individuals with AK-47s. Request permission to engage.'

Pilot: 'Light 'em all up!'

Their voices take me back to the palace, put me in front of that small, boxy TV monitor. So does the hellish rhythmic clack of Crazy Horse 1–8's chain gun. I breathe deeply to counter the anxiety in my chest. I watch the video again, this time taking notes. And again. I'll watch the footage dozens of times over the coming weeks, checking and rechecking details, timings to the second. But it isn't as hard as I thought. I'll conclude it's because I've made peace with Namir and Saeed and myself over what happened in Baghdad on 12 July 2007.

PART THREE

15

Inferno

I answer the incoming Skype call from a Reuters colleague who has asked to talk. They want to remain anonymous because they still work at Reuters. I suspect they will tell their story one day, when it's right for them. For now, I will refer to them as DZ. But I look forward to shouting from the rooftops the name of this young person who taught me that *everyone* who has suffered trauma belongs to the same community. That we can *all* learn from each other, no matter what we went through.

Until I spoke to DZ, I wasn't sure what to say to a sexual assault survivor. I could put myself in the shoes of soldiers, first responders and medical teams, victims of natural disasters and road accidents, even civilians in warzones if I tried hard enough. But not survivors of sexual assault. I've never been raped or sexually abused. I couldn't begin to imagine carrying that violence around in my head, my body. To be honest, I don't think I wanted to try because it was too horrific.

I also thought survivors would only want to share such trauma with a clinician, a close friend or family. While I was pushing hard to normalise the conversation around mental illness at Reuters – my role had been broadened from PTSD advocate to encompass mental health more broadly – I wasn't saying or doing anything to address sexual assault and harassment in the organisation. I didn't think I belonged in that space because I was male. I also have no experience of personal harassment of any kind.

I know something is wrong as soon as DZ says hello. DZ sits stiffly, back pressed into a chair, a pained look on their face. It hasn't been easy for DZ to contact a stranger, a man. DZ looks only a few years out of university. It's 31 May 2018.

'How can I help?' I ask.

DZ says a much older male colleague raped them seven months ago in a hotel not far from the capital of the country where they are based. DZ was working on a story at the time. An HR executive investigated last month but dismissed the complaint because of 'inconclusive' evidence. DZ contacted me because they didn't know who else to turn to.

DZ has spoken quietly, their emotions mostly under control.

I am so sorry, I say. I tell DZ I believe them and ask if they would feel comfortable sharing more of their story. I'm not a counsellor, I say, but I can help staff navigate HR and management bureaucracy. In my role as head of mental health and wellbeing strategy, I know how to escalate issues and to whom.

DZ closes their eyes briefly, then begins.

How this man groomed DZ is not my story to share. I'll only say that I suspect he saw a bright but vulnerable journalist in their first media job when he approached DZ to collaborate on stories. He offered to mentor his young colleague, who was married.

In the weeks that followed, DZ repeatedly said no to an intimate or romantic relationship but felt trapped by the man's persistence and mentoring.

A few weeks later, he turned up at DZ's hotel one night outside the city where DZ was working, drank too much to drive back and asked to sleep in DZ's room. It was an industrial town. No other hotel was within walking distance. DZ said he could stay but only if he understood they did not want to have sex.

The first time the man penetrated them, DZ froze, unable to move or speak. He didn't wear a condom. When he raped DZ a second time, again without a condom, DZ repeatedly said 'no' and 'please stop'. He stopped only when DZ began to cry, then got angry. He shouted and punched a pillow. Afraid he'd get violent beyond the rape, DZ decided to have sex to calm him. DZ pretended to enjoy it.

DZ didn't go to the police because the country where the rape occurred offers little legal protection to sexual assault survivors. Shame stopped DZ reporting the rape to Reuters until a senior editor who had hired DZ happened to visit months later. In a catch-up meeting, DZ broke down and told him briefly what had happened. He alerted the HR executive with DZ's consent. Several days later, the HR executive interviewed DZ in a hotel cafe for 90 minutes. No one else was present. Nor was the interview recorded and the executive barely took notes. The HR executive asked DZ to go to the newsroom later that day for a second interview which lasted twenty minutes. It wasn't recorded either. A week later, DZ was diagnosed with PTSD.

The following day, the HR executive told DZ by phone that the complaint had been dismissed due to inconclusive evidence. Sobbing, and after much back and forth, DZ expressed fear about returning to work. Reuters could make reasonable adjustments but if DZ couldn't be in the same newsroom as the male colleague, who'd been suspended during the investigation but was now free to go back, the HR executive said, 'maybe you have to leave'. DZ curled up on the floor of their apartment for a couple of hours, then recorded an audio suicide note, called their partner at his office to say goodbye and tried to kill themselves. DZ's partner arrived home just in time.

I've listened to DZ's recording. Even now, years later, I'm lost for words to describe the darkness and isolation that had engulfed DZ. The anguish and bewilderment at not being believed.

I again tell DZ how sorry I am. I'm shocked Reuters didn't believe you, I say. Being interviewed in a coffee shop with no support person present was unprofessional and could have retraumatised you. I urge DZ to write to the global head of HR in New York and explain in detail the rapes, the PTSD diagnosis, the way HR handled it and the impact all this has had on their mental health. I suspect New York knows the outlines but little else.

'I thought this decision would be final,' DZ says, surprised.

'No, you can bypass these people. I'll help you.'

I explain that I can connect DZ with the company's 24/7 global trauma support service. I pause, then gently ask if DZ feels suicidal now. DZ says no – they have a good therapist. I ask if they know of the Reuters peer network, the group of journalists trained to support colleagues in distress. The HR executive never suggested it and DZ hasn't heard of it. With DZ's approval, as soon as we finish talking, I call a senior peer, a veteran and empathic journalist in London, who contacts DZ within hours.

*

My stomach churns with disgust at Reuters. Leaving this young journalist to rot in their apartment for six weeks, knowing DZ is too frightened to return to work. Reuters might not know DZ attempted suicide, but anyone with a basic understanding of trauma would know self-harm was a risk. Now there is the added complication of the PTSD diagnosis. It will be nearly two years before DZ gets back to work for Reuters, in a country on the other side of the world.

DZ was raped in late October 2017. Earlier that month, the *New York Times* and the *New Yorker* magazine reported widespread sexual abuse allegations against Harvey Weinstein. Within a week, the hashtag #MeToo went viral on social media, unleashing a long overdue reckoning in global workplaces. Women came forward with accounts of sexual assault and harassment in film, fashion, car manufacturing, finance, politics, music, hospitality and of course the media industry. People from other marginalised groups spoke up. Survivors were believed. Men were investigated and fired. Except, it seemed, at Reuters.

In a text message the next day, DZ says that writing to the head of HR is proving cathartic: 'I finally feel I'm not alone in this company.'

'Let me know how it goes,' I reply. 'I won't hesitate to intervene if necessary, you have my word.'

—

DZ is the latest in a string of colleagues to contact me since my mental health role was announced a year ago. It wasn't long before Reuters journalists came to me, seeking advice, saying managers were harming their mental health.

Around the time DZ reaches out, a former Reuters journalist

tells me via Facebook that she thinks about dying every day. I'm familiar with her work in dangerous places and unaware she has left the company. She had been a high-flyer. I ask if she is suicidal. She says she is okay now but tried to kill herself a few months earlier. She developed PTSD from years of covering traumatic stories for Reuters as well as from childhood sexual abuse. She quit after being put on a performance improvement plan, believing she'd be fired. She regretted not being open with Reuters about her PTSD. I put her in touch with the trauma support service, which is available to alumni.

Another colleague asks if I can check on a friend of hers, a former Reuters journalist also suffering PTSD from reporting in warzones. She is worried about his welfare. This man tells me he can't work because of his condition. 'I'm really stuck. I'm aimless. It's horrible not being able to work.'

A senior manager tells me she questions whether she and other editors did enough to help a Reuters journalist who had been fired because of drunkenness at work. The sacked woman was diagnosed with PTSD a few weeks later.

The anger from when Reuters was indifferent to me in 2016, saw me as damaged goods and tried to force me out, still flows through my veins. I want people held accountable.

Adding to my growing rage, QBE, Reuters' workers' compensation insurer, has told me it's disputing a claim I've made for PTSD-related medical expenses. HR had asked me to claim the cost of my second Ward 17 admission as well as out-patient psych bills through the insurer. I was fine with this because it was purely about expenses. I lodged an initial claim via HR in Sydney in December 2017. QBE then spent five months combing through my medical and employment history.

I dial into a telephone hearing with the Tasmanian Workers

Rehabilitation and Compensation Tribunal on 5 June, less than a week after my first conversation with DZ. During the hearing, a lawyer for QBE acknowledges that I am 'suffering from a significant disease' but says Tasmania has no connection to my trauma exposure overseas and that I filed the claim too late. QBE is not liable.

I argue with the tribunal's chief commissioner. I call the process 'ethically and morally reprehensible' but he rules in favour of QBE. I can appeal if I want, he says. Luckily, I wasn't in the workers' comp system, with QBE paying my salary, because the commissioner would have stopped that immediately. Reuters keeps paying the psych bills. An HR rep from Sydney is on the phone but says nothing.

A tiny part of the brain called the amygdala decides in an instant what to do when someone is confronted with a potential life threat – fight, flight or freeze. A fourth response gaining acceptance is called fawn, which describes often unconscious behaviour to placate an attacker. When raped, people usually don't fight back or scream for help. They freeze. In the scientific community this is known as tonic immobility, or a state of paralysis. A Swedish study published in 2017 showed that 70 per cent of 298 women at a Stockholm clinic for rape survivors reported significant tonic immobility and 48 per cent extreme tonic immobility during their assault. The research team found that having experienced tonic immobility more than doubled the chance of PTSD at the six-month follow-up and the likelihood of severe depression threefold. Courts may be inclined to dismiss rape because a survivor didn't appear to resist, the study said. Instead, what might be interpreted as passive consent was very likely the normal and expected biological reactions to an overwhelming threat.

Reuters and other foreign media wrote stories on the landmark Swedish research. I send a link to DZ. It helps DZ understand why they froze during the first rape.

For now, in the days after our initial conversation, I suggest DZ might find *Trauma and Recovery* by American psychiatrist Judith Herman and *The Body Keeps the Score* by Bessel van der Kolk useful. *Trauma and Recovery* was hailed as ground-breaking when it was published in 1992. Herman drew on two decades of her research and clinical work with survivors of sexual assault and domestic violence as well as the experiences of other traumatised people such as combat veterans and survivors of political terror.

It was only when I read Herman's book during my first Ward 17 admission that I got a proper insight into what rape does to women and the social context in which it occurs. It had taken me 47 years, and it was because I was searching for understanding into my own crisis. I was a well-travelled foreign correspondent, I'd read widely, I knew a lot of women. But I lived life in a man's bubble. I didn't really see or sense the violence perpetrated by men on half the world's population.

DZ sends me essays on female rage and pain by feminist authors such as Audre Lorde. I send DZ blogs I've written about PTSD and moral injury. DZ seeks my advice on the complaint they are writing for the head of HR. We talk about the #MeToo Movement, trying to understand how Reuters existed in a different universe when it investigated DZ's initial complaint. We also talk about our journeys, discovering we have much in common: flashbacks, nightmares and chest-crushing anxiety; we are both in therapy and on medication; and betrayal by Reuters, we share that too.

After DZ emails the global head of HR, I also message her. I want the New York office to know that I know. I've seen

DZ's complaint. I'm shocked and horrified by what DZ has gone through, I write, and about their isolation within Reuters. The HR chief assures me Reuters is responding fairly and appropriately.

DZ prepares well for their first call with the head of HR. They are determined to try to fix the company's complaints process and policies and procedures on sexual harassment and assault. The head of HR tells DZ that Reuters will hire a prominent foreign legal practitioner who specialises in sexual harassment in the workplace to investigate DZ's accusations.

DZ is not sure what to think. 'It's a good outcome,' I say. 'You're being taken seriously.' I suggest DZ work on a timeline of events, adding I'd be happy to review it, but understand if they keep it private because of the deeply personal information.

'Despite what I try to tell myself, I still feel ashamed and implicated in what happened, and it's hard to share details with other people, especially someone I respect,' DZ says in an email.

'I won't judge you,' I reply. 'Ever. I know what it feels like to feel shame. It affected me for years after the deaths of my staff in Baghdad. In my personal life, I have done things I'm ashamed of. But I now have more self-compassion. That has helped me deal with these things.'

DZ writes back: 'Whenever I read other women's accounts of harassment and rape, I never think they are implicated, but somehow, when it comes to my own story, it's hard to find compassion. There's always a nagging sense I'm morally or ethically worse than other victims of rape, and therefore I am more responsible for what happened.'

It will take DZ a long time to accept that like virtually every story of sexual harassment and rape, theirs is messy and complicated too.

DZ spends the next few weeks working on the timeline, reading, journaling and reflecting. One day DZ has a revelation about inconclusive evidence, words that locked them into an 'impossible, endless obsession with proof'.

'As you pointed out, #MeToo is about believing, not proving,' DZ writes to me. 'The language of "evidence" made me forget that fact and displaced me from the narrative of #MeToo – I wasn't battling to be believed, as #MeToo women were. I was battling to *prove*, which in my case was impossible. I stopped reading #MeToo stories because they seemed to exist in an alternate world to which I had no access. #MeToo victims lived in a world of believability; I lived in a world of evidence.

'I kept questioning myself: What is "conclusive" evidence? Do I have "conclusive" evidence? Would I lose again since I clearly lack "conclusive" evidence? That is why I have been doubting the validity and importance of my timeline: it is, after all, just my memories and interpretations. But finally, with the help of Judith Herman, I ventured out of my cage and read the #MeToo stories I was afraid to read. This is what I needed, to see myself as part of #MeToo. To imagine myself being heard, being believed, being vindicated. To realise that all I have is my words and memories, and that is enough.'

DZ has also got me thinking about something I said recently. That I felt it wasn't my place to get involved in sexual harassment issues at Reuters despite my mental health role, because I was a man. I'd given the issue some thought. I'd always assumed Mary contended with lecherous old editors and sexism as a young journalist in Tasmania in the 1980s. But I didn't know how bad it was until the #MeToo Movement and Mary told me about her experiences: how as a young reporter an older journalist groomed her into having a relationship. On another occasion after she had dinner with an interstate journalist a few years older than her at his home, he blocked the door when she went to leave, got angry and demanded sex. Frightened by his aggression, Mary 'got it over with' so she could leave. Years later, after we were married, a colleague asked Mary to perform a sex act on him. When she refused, he said: 'I could rape you.'

I was horrified. My brave partner, my beacon of inspiration, being preyed upon by evil men. Mary wouldn't tell me who the colleague was or which country they were in when he threatened her, but I know the names of the other two. I also know the name of DZ's rapist.

DZ was surprised when I said I wouldn't get involved in sexual harassment issues at Reuters. They hadn't even thought about my gender until I raised it.

'This is strange, since I've been religiously avoiding male therapists and male psychiatrists and male anyone who wasn't family. The fact you suffered and survived trauma trumped all else; I saw you as someone who has gone through the hell that I went through. The fact you are male was irrelevant. You are in an extremely special and powerful position because creating strategies and policies surrounding mental health is your role . . . You have the ears of people who have the power to effect structural change – you can do and say things that others in the company cannot.'

DZ gets me thinking about how quick I am to tell people to avoid comparing their trauma or mental illness to someone else: get into the comparison game and you play down your symptoms, miss out on help, I say. I've been unable to kick the comparison with sexual assault survivors until now. Judith Herman in the introduction of *Trauma and Recovery* writes about commonalities 'between rape survivors and combat veterans, between battered women and political prisoners, between the survivors of vast concentration camps created by tyrants who rule nations and the survivors of small, hidden concentration camps created by tyrants who rule their homes'. DZ helped me see how true that is.

—

It's now mid-July. DZ hasn't worked for more than three months; DZ's male colleague isn't being suspended during the appeal process; DZ's hypervigilance and anxiety make it difficult to go outside, be around men. Attending therapy is hard enough. DZ sleeps poorly, tries to devote energy to the timeline and prepare for the interview with the investigator, who will fly to DZ's location in early August. Reuters says DZ can have a support person on the phone. DZ wants their peer colleague from London in the room, but Reuters refuses to pay. When I tell the global head of HR I'm going to get on a plane to attend the interview, Reuters agrees to cover the colleague's travel costs.

DZ was a red line and I suspect the global head of HR knew that.

The more I talk and exchange messages with DZ, the more I obsess over the way I was treated in 2016. It's a betrayal that has left a festering wound. My new boss and the head of HR have been wonderfully supportive, both of me and my family. But for the mental health campaign at Reuters to mean anything, I need to set the standard in holding the company to account. It's not enough to help colleagues such as DZ, so I decide to file a formal complaint about what happened to me.

I begin work on a 20,000-word timeline and a 3000-word

statement setting out how I believe certain individuals breached the company's code of conduct by failing to act ethically and with transparency. Jeremy Wagstaff, his partner Sari Sudarsono and their daughter Charlotte, and Tessa Piper arrive for their annual visit to Evandale around this time. Jeremy and I walk around the village each morning after dawn, then sit at the kitchen table in front of our laptops. Jeremy is writing a book. I work on my timeline.

One evening, I'm in front of the wood-fired heater when Jeremy, Sari and Tessa sit near me. Mary pulls up a chair. It's an ambush. With Jeremy taking the lead, they say the complaint is a bad idea. It might jeopardise the ambitious goals I have for my mental health agenda at Reuters and burn the bridges I've spent eighteen months trying to build. It's also draining me when I should be relaxing on holiday. I agree to shelve the complaint and move on. Secretly, I keep working on it. I can't let it go; the betrayal is too deep.

I lie in bed at night, fixated. My nightmares return after a period without any. I wake with bags under my eyes. Most afternoons I need to sleep. I jump out of my skin at unexpected noise and tense up inside supermarkets or cafes. When our friends fly home, I drink heavily, sometimes in the morning. I need Valium every day. DZ's timeline drafts make my blood boil. Mary and the kids are walking on eggshells again.

In early August, Mary urges me to go back to Ward 17, saying some of my symptoms are as bad as before my first admission. To her relief, I don't argue. I'm self-aware enough to know I'm on the brink.

I email my psychologist Wendy Gall asking for a referral. 'I'm feeling pretty explosive,' I write. 'All I want to watch is revenge movies. I'm listening to angry music.'

I also email Dr Maryam, asking if she can look after me again.

'The root cause of all this is multiple layers of anger towards the Reuters people who never supported me in the first place, the fact I'm fighting QBE without any support, and the sheer number of Reuters journalists who have turned to me for help because they have been so badly treated,' I say.

I write to my boss, saying I need another admission to Ward 17. I send him the complaint informally. Fuck it, Reuters needs to know.

I'm not having flashbacks, and I don't think my depression is too bad, though Mary disagrees. I'm not numb to my kids like in the years leading up to 2016. Anger is the real worry. I was angry in 2016, but not like this.

When Mary gets home from work the next day, I'm feeling more stable. I've just gotten a tattoo on my left shoulder. It shows the PTSD teal ribbon. Inside are the words Iraq, Aceh and Bali. I'm excited to show Mary. I've cooked dinner for myself and the kids, but forgotten about Mary, who is now vegetarian. She asks if there is anything for her. I erupt. She has never seen such anger on my face in our 23 years together.

DZ, meanwhile, has just finished two rounds of interviews with the investigator, sixteen hours in total, and is exhausted. The investigator wants to do more but had to fly home for other commitments. I don't tell DZ I'm going back to Ward 17.

Later that month, DZ is in a city far from home before the final interview with the investigator. I'm preparing to fly to Melbourne. DZ now knows my third Ward 17 admission is coming up.

'We are both at new stages of our fights. I know we will both come out stronger and with more wisdom,' DZ says in an email.

'Absolutely, different stages of our fights but same resolve!' I reply.

16

Awakening

Fear consumed me when I entered Ward 17 two years ago. I was in disbelief trudging past the Diggers Way road-sign last year. This time is different; I want to be admitted. My anger scares me. I'm just not sure how Ward 17 will help.

It's Thursday, 23 August 2018. I caught an early flight from Launceston and arrived at Ward 17 just after breakfast. I'm wearing blue jeans, a brown woollen jumper, black coat and my R.M. Williams boots. Overdressed again but I don't care. Admission is easy, I know the drill. I don't recognise any patients, but it doesn't matter. I introduce myself to those near the nurse's station before I'm taken to Room 13. My previous rooms, 11 and 15, are in the same corridor. I open the door to Room 15 by mistake a few times over the coming days. Luckily, it's empty. Returning to Ward 17 is like slipping on an old shoe.

Dr Maryam sees me within an hour, which makes me want to hug her (I don't).

I'm in the usual patient–therapist room with Maryam and a

psychiatry registrar and a nurse. I'd given Maryam some background in my email two weeks ago.

'Are you feeling suicidal?' Maryam asks

I shake my head. I'm too angry.

My boss is trying to arrange for the global head of HR to brief me on what happened in 2016, I say. Maryam expresses concern about me doing this in Ward 17 while I'm enraged. I counter by saying I need the supported environment should the conversation go badly. We talk about explanations I can live with. Maryam suggests I write them down over the weekend.

I tell Maryam about DZ and other colleagues who've sought my help since my new job was announced fifteen months ago, the pain and betrayal they carry from management. I take Maryam through a submission I'm writing for a federal senate inquiry into the high rates of mental illness among first responders. I'm explaining how easy it is for insurance companies to stop making wage and medical payments to police and emergency service personnel, using the data I have for Tasmania. While the terms of reference don't include the media, journalists who cover traumatic events are first responders, I've written. They rush to accidents, natural disasters and terrorist attacks and can be exposed to trauma while reporting on court trials and crime.

What I've become more concerned about in my role at Reuters is distressing imagery – the risk of vicarious trauma from viewing and editing images of war, violence and suffering. The *DSM-5* says professionals such as journalists can develop PTSD from repeated exposure to distressing material.

Maryam knows what motivates me and why I'm angry. She also knows this is hurting my recovery and says so.

'But how do I reconcile this with the person I want to be? This is what drives me,' I say.

'You can't fight battles on multiple fronts when you have PTSD,' Maryam replies.

I think Maryam senses I'm riled up, not ready to compromise. I drank my last rum and coke only eight or nine hours ago. She shifts the conversation to self-care. Use the time in Ward 17 to get your routine back on track, she says. We can agree on that. I've resolved to start walking daily again, followed by 60 sit-ups and meditation. I want to lose weight. She orders me not to do any Reuters work. Fine, I say.

We talk about my nightmares. Interestingly, I'm not having flashbacks, though I started getting very depressed a few days ago. This worries Maryam, so she increases my Pristiq to 150 mg a day from 100 mg, adding I might need to go to 200 mg, a heavy dose. She calls this my third bout of major depressive disorder, which means I might need to stay on antidepressants for five to ten years, which doesn't bother me. Higher dosages could help my anxiety and anger, something I wasn't aware of. It's not that you can't be depressed when you're angry. But anger can muffle other symptoms.

It's a relief getting things off my chest with Maryam. But back in my room I wonder how she can help given that everything hinges on the head of HR. Later that day my assigned nurse drops by. We'd have fewer patients here if organisations took care of their staff, she says with a tired look.

'But you have to own your anger. You're responsible for that, not HR,' she adds. 'And you must establish clear boundaries with colleagues. You're not a clinician.' I like it how the nurses speak their minds.

Patients share their stories with me over dinner. One is Stewart Hulls, an affable former copper from Maryborough in country

Victoria who is a few years younger than me. Stewart investigated fatal collisions for highway patrol based out of a small town for fifteen years. He knew five of the people whose accidents he investigated. Three were good friends. Stewart has a long-term back injury and walks with a limp from his own motorcycle accident the previous year. He was diagnosed with PTSD in 2014 and has fought the police's insurance company for compensation ever since. The stress and frustration of that battle is one reason Stewart is here on his first admission.

In late 2021, Stewart will tell me he eventually got a payout of $240,000 for his physical injuries. For his PTSD, zero. Nothing, after four and a half years of seeking compensation. 'It was never about the money, just what was fair,' he says. 'I think they try to wear you down because they know you've got a mental injury. They want you to walk away. Otherwise, why should it take so long? When you have to fight like this, it takes away all your coping mechanisms for dealing with PTSD. You're almost ready to bite the bullet.'

Stewart loved his job despite the trauma. He said he'd have been fine if the insurer took several months to check his claim for PTSD and content with a fair lump sum over his mental state. And he wanted recognition from Victoria Police that he left the force because PTSD had broken him. Sounds reasonable to me. Instead, his bosses hung him out to dry and then the workers' comp system crushed him.

—

I routinely speak to my manager in New York every Friday morning. He emails overnight asking if I want to settle in to Ward 17 instead. I reply, saying I still want to talk:

215

'As I said to my psychiatrist yesterday, until I get an explanation of what happened in 2016 and why, everything I do here won't have a lasting effect on my mental state. The folks here can prop me up. But they have seen rage like mine before, they know it can kill a person's chances of recovery. I need the truth. Only then can I do the work I need to do to move on.'

Later, on the phone, my boss tells me he doesn't know exactly what happened, but believes there might have been some miscommunication and that no one ever said, 'Let's get rid of that Dean Yates.'

'I suspect there were concerns about whether you could do the [mentoring] job, a feeling we needed to rethink the whole thing – as in the new job,' he says.

Really, I think to myself, why didn't someone just say that? I would have understood if Reuters had come to me after my first Ward 17 discharge two years ago and said: 'Dean, we're worried about whether you can handle this new role, let's talk through all the options.' Had I been treated with dignity and respect, offered an honourable exit with a good settlement, I probably would have signed.

Reuters knew how fragile I was because I reacted so badly to the 12 October phone conversation when Reece first cast doubt on the mentoring role. Reece even acknowledged this had caused me 'significant stress'. Despite this, despite knowing I'd left Ward 17 only a month earlier, Reuters went ahead with actions that might have made me harm myself, and which at a minimum derailed my recovery and threatened my family's future.

Australian trauma clinicians Zachary Steel and Dominic Hilbrink wrote in 2015 of their work with veterans and emergency service personnel at the St John of God psychiatric hospital near Sydney. They said that soldiers and first responders could often cope with high stress and traumatic exposure if they had an organisational and social structure behind them. But moral injury could occur if superiors failed to provide crucial support when it was most needed. This betrayal could be experienced as an attack on the self that is 'every bit as real and visceral as a physical threat', they wrote.

Steel, also a professor in trauma and mental health at the School of Psychiatry at the University of New South Wales, told me he'd seen many veterans and first responders struggle because of poor organisational support. They had training and experience to prepare for and accommodate 'life threat', as opposed to moral injury which is much harder to train for and may often occur due to systemic organisational failure.

Jonathan Shay says something similar: where 'leadership malpractice inflicts moral injury, the body codes it as a physical attack, mobilises for danger and counterattack, and lastingly imprints the physiology every bit as much as if it had been a physical attack'.

———

I'm depressed, tired and shaky. My thoughts are scattered, unlike the laser focus I had during previous admissions. I'm in a holding pattern. My boss gives no timeframe for when I can talk to the head of HR and I can't be bothered drawing up explanations I might get. Mary is writing to Maryam but doesn't want me to see her email. Have I sacrificed my family to help my colleagues?

I'd emailed spiritual care worker Cath Taylor a week before my admission and had a chat with her soon after I arrived. I suspect Cath holds the key. Cath runs a group session on meaning and values on Monday morning. I'll see her again that afternoon.

About seven or eight patients attend. Cath gives us each an A3 sheet of paper with 120 values written on them. That's a lot, I think. 'Scan the page and choose ten you hold most dearly,' Cath says. 'Don't think too hard, trust your instincts.'

Cath gives us a few minutes to write each value on a separate yellow post-it note. My eyes lock on the first one – accountability. I also choose compassion, empathy, fairness, honesty, justice, making a difference, sensitivity, tolerance and truth-seeking. Cath asks us to remove three, then another three. My remaining four are:

Accountability

Honesty

Empathy

Justice

Cath gives us a blank A3 piece of paper and asks us to write what each value means to us and how we express it in daily life. I write:

Accountability
- *It's devastating when there is no accountability.*
- *Make the company accountable for what was done to me.*
- *Fight for a Truth and Reconciliation Commission at Reuters.*

Honesty
- *Without honesty there is no trust.*
- *No secrets with anyone.*
- *Encourage managers to be more honest.*
- *Total transparency.*

Justice
- *There is so much injustice, it's infuriating.*

218

> – *FIGHT, Fight for changes in legislation. Fight insurance companies. Fight for strong mental health workplace policies.*

Empathy
> – *I find it easy to have empathy for others who are suffering.*
> – *I open myself to others.*
> – *Educate Reuters about the importance of empathy.*

We go round the table. A veteran and a copper, both men, speak first. Their values are like mine. I lean forward, right foot tapping, when it's my turn. Then a female prison guard next to me says her first value is love. My heart sinks. I look at the list of values on the A3 sheet. I hadn't seen the word. I'm silent for the rest of the session.

Later that day, Cath and I sit in the small corner TV room. Cath is eighteen weeks pregnant, expecting her first child and looks radiant. I tell her she will make an awesome mum. Maryam and social worker Christina Sim have both been firm with me in Ward 17, occasionally tough. I don't think it's in Cath's nature – she is the spiritual care worker – but she doesn't hold back.

'Dean – what was going on this morning? Your values were all about the mistreatment of yourself and your colleagues. There was nothing about love or family.'

'Was there a value about family?' I ask, eyes wide.

'Family-oriented,' Cath replies.

'I didn't see it. I'm just so enveloped in anger,' I say, looking up at the ceiling.

I once asked Mary what has been my most destructive trauma symptom. Rage, she said without missing a beat.

*

Cath tells me a parable about a Zen master and his apprentice walking along a track. They come to a stream where an old woman is waiting. The Zen master picks her up and carries her to the other side. The woman moves off without saying a word, leaving the apprentice speechless. An hour passes without conversation. Two hours, three.

The young monk blurts out: 'Aren't you angry she didn't thank you?'

The master looks at him and says: 'Brother, I'm not carrying her anymore, why are you?'

'Have I lost all perspective?' I ask Cath.

'I wouldn't call it that,' she says. 'The question is, are you waiting for this outcome or are you living life irrespective of it? I can feel this wall of anger around you. There is no softness.'

I wonder if that's why Mary wants to send a private email to Maryam. She's scared of my reaction. At home I've been going to bed early, thinking of revenge. Mary stays in the living room, alone, watching TV. I've shut my family out because of this anger, I say.

'How long have you been like this?'

'Weeks. But it's been bubbling for a long time.'

—

Back in my room I sit in the green armchair, remove my shoes, put my feet on the bed. I like seeing the same gum trees through the large window.

Everyone runs into dead-ends, goes round in circles in their struggle to heal from trauma. There are also turning points. Today is a Big One but it will take time – like years – for me to realise this.

What I sense right now is that sharing my story will communalise my trauma. Help me heal.

What's more important? Fighting my own battle or putting in place policies at Reuters that will stop it happening to others? Should I let it go?

I call Mary, asking if she thinks I've gotten things out of perspective. I think she agrees but doesn't want to say so directly.

I ask my friend Jeremy Wagstaff on WhatsApp the same question. He replies: 'You are in a completely different place. You have protection from the highest levels at Reuters. A sense of mission. A treating team at Ward 17. You understand so much more about PTSD. In 2016 we were in a bunker. The idea of not pursuing the complaint was a good one. But if it's troubling you, I can understand if you won't let it go. It was an injustice. The chronology is seared into our minds.'

Ward 17 is clearing my head. But it's not like flipping a switch. My body doesn't work that way. The next day I wake about 3.30 am and toss and turn. A few hours later I can't get out of bed for my walk. I'm depressed. I'm making progress intellectually, but my body is stuck.

The word *obsession* slips out of my mouth in my next session with Maryam, who nearly leaps out of her chair.

'Yes!' she exclaims. 'You're obsessed with these things and look at what it's doing to you and your family.'

Maryam talks about a table made of compressed glass that she owns. At some point, it must have developed a hairline crack. She and her husband had moved recently. One night they were sitting near the table when a shard of glass shot into the air.

'You are that compressed glass. That's your anger,' she says.

I tell Maryam I've started to question whether I need an

explanation of what happened in 2016. 'Exactly,' she says. 'What difference would it make?'

'But I still want to expose how QBE treated me.'

'Why put so much effort into this?' Maryam asks.

'Because I can make a difference, use my skills as a journalist.'

'What's the end game?'

I tell her that I don't care whether I'm successful or not, I just want to draw attention to how these insurance companies operate.

Maryam says I need to learn to read my emotions each day. My emotions and body are way behind my cognitive understanding of my obsession, she believes. She suggests I set goals for each week and month and bring those goals into balance with family life. Don't be focused on doing, doing, doing.

'I'm pleased with your progress,' Maryam says.

'Do I get a tick?'

'A half tick,' she says with a smile.

Mary sends her email to Maryam a couple of hours later, then forwards it to me.

Hi Maryam,

I hope you enjoyed your time off with your little one. Thanks so much for all you're doing for Dean. You are a shining beacon for us. Dean said you would be interested in my observations of his symptoms prior to his admission. I was reluctant to do this at first because emotionally it's terribly hard to do – especially as it hurts Dean – but I must for all those families affected by PTSD . . .

We had an incident of anger in which I felt very frightened because it was so out of character. I'd come home to the children having had takeaway but nothing I could eat. It wasn't really that there wasn't anything for me – I can look after myself – but the crushing disappointment of feeling I was absolutely powerless to stop Dean's descent. On this occasion, Dean had talked obsessively about the latest injustices at Reuters – and I don't underplay the seriousness of them – but they were gaining more importance than our family. I sat numbly until Dean asked me what was wrong. I said there was nothing for me to eat. It sounded selfish, I know, but it was just symptomatic of the situation. I felt despair and a sense of loneliness. The anger was different to the episode I experienced before Dean's first admission to hospital where I felt I needed to walk away before he hit me. This time it was a deep, seething and threatening anger. I didn't know what to do. I knew that to confront him would make things worse, so I backed down to avoid any escalation. I felt I didn't know this person, and that even when he was talking to me, it wasn't me he was talking to.

Dean became obsessed with other people's injustices at Reuters, which fuelled and triggered his own anger at how he'd been treated. I don't take anything away from the tremendous trauma these people suffered, but they were living in our house, they were virtually tangible. The children and I were ghosts. Yes, Dean would do anything for us – he ferried Harry to the gym every night and would do anything for our other children – but I felt we weren't there. Or maybe he wasn't with us. The obsession with other people's cases triggered his own trauma, sent him to bed frequently and deprived us of a normal family life. I think somehow Dean needed to lose himself in these cases, but I could see that it was making him re-live his own trauma.

Since my mother died recently I've had a persistent feeling of grieving alone, and have resented this, although I now understand in hindsight that Dean didn't have the mental capacity to deal with my grief. I've had to take my father, 87, under my wing, but I've felt

Dean's absence, and this too has hurt, but once again I know he just hasn't had the bandwidth. I suppose what I'm saying is that isolation can destroy relationships.

I'm terribly sorry, Maryam, if I sound selfish or have outlined Dean's symptoms in the context of how they have affected me. I know that when Dean reads this – and I know it helps him if he does – I'll feel I've kicked him when he's down. But PTSD is so destructive of families, and I will do anything to save mine.

I'm glad Mary shared the email with me. As well as writing about my anger and obsession, Mary outlined a dozen other symptoms such as nightmares, noise sensitivity, fatigue and an unwillingness to change my clothes. I feel a bit hurt, but everything is true, although I'd tried to argue I was reducing the washing by wearing the same clothes.

I have been emotionally absent for Mary since the death of her mother a few months ago and that was wrong.

It was like Mary described: she and the children were ghosts. Anger dominated, not love, not family.

All the pieces have fallen into place. I send my manager an email, saying I don't need an explanation for what happened in 2016. I call Mary to tell her. I apologise for being so obsessed at the expense of her and the kids.

—

While I've made a major decision, my body doesn't feel relieved. My nervous system has been in a state of heightened arousal for months. I'm depressed and tired. Even teary. I sleep badly.

I stay in Ward 17 for another two weeks, getting my routine back on track. I walk every day for 45 minutes then do 60 sit-ups.

I attend a daily 9 am mindfulness session. I meditate on my bed for twenty minutes. I've also taken up Tai Chi with a former naval submariner called Adrian Jallands, who, like me, loves rugby league and is in a room a couple of doors along. We watch every game each weekend in the corner TV room.

I do more group and individual work with my treating team. In one group session, OT Michelle talks about the window of tolerance, sensory modulation and arousal regulation. On a whiteboard, Michelle writes the following:

Signs of Hyper-arousal:
  - *Emotional, overwhelmed, panic, impulsive, hypervigilance, defensiveness, feeling unsafe, reactive, irritable, racing thoughts.*

Window of Tolerance (Optimal Level):
  - *Feelings and reactions are tolerable; we can think and feel simultaneously; our reactions adapt to fit the situation.*

Signs of Hypo-arousal:
  - *Numb, passive, no feelings, no energy, cannot think, feeling disconnected, 'not there', shut down.*

When you wake each morning, work out your baseline level, Michelle says. Are you within your window of tolerance? To stay inside or to get back in, practise calming strategies. You can't regulate yourself if you don't know where you sit on the spectrum.

'Set your intention to do this. It's your promise to yourself,' Michelle says.

Social worker Christina Sim suggests I mentally check my window of tolerance three times a day. She calls the exercise 'deliberate self-awareness', being able to modify my arousal levels to stay in my window of tolerance.

It feels good to have stopped obsessing about 2016. I decide I also need to ring-fence myself from the trauma of my colleagues and tell Maryam I'll set boundaries. Maryam says when she meets people in a social setting, they sometimes talk about personal matters after finding out she is a psychiatrist. 'Here, I'm Maryam, not your doctor,' is what she politely tells them.

Maryam says she wants me to work with Wendy Gall on anger management and see her regularly when I get home. I've had only four appointments with Wendy in the past eight months. I like and respect Wendy, but I think I've avoided making routine appointments (even though Reuters pays) because I don't have the Ward 17 guardrails around me. I'm afraid of getting too deep into an issue outside these safe walls. It sounds counterintuitive, but Maryam says the most important time for therapy is when I'm good because that lays a foundation to nip a crisis in the bud. She says she has seldom seen a patient with PTSD who didn't have anger problems. This is not always directed at employers and insurance companies, which is common in Ward 17 given the nature of the place. People can be angry at the world, at themselves. She sees anger more in men. They can be frightened of themselves and withdraw. In this 'silent anger', men ignore others, don't communicate at the height of their rage.

'Can you now understand how your anger affected Mary?' Maryam asks.

'Yes. I can put myself in her shoes. It would have been terrifying.'

'You need to recognise when you are getting angry or anxious and bring yourself down. Know your red flags. Look in the mirror. See what you look like.'

I write a lot over the following weekend. I'm getting a deeper understanding of how hard I was to live with. Also, that I did this self-awareness and self-regulation work with Michelle during my first admission two years ago! I'd either forgotten everything or not revised it. I'd taped small cards to the bottom of my computer monitor at home after my first admission with tips on regulating anger and anxiety. But other items on my desk obscured the cards and I haven't looked at them since. I'll later take them off the monitor, put each one in my printer and make larger copies and stick them on my noticeboard.

I tell Christina that being back in Ward 17 has made me realise how much I love Mary and want to start a new chapter with her. I've realised how destructive going to sex workers was to our relationship. I was selfish and I'm ashamed of that. I want to understand Mary's wishes, needs and desires. I want to be the best possible husband and father I can be. Christina is delighted when I say Mary has agreed to renew our vows under the walnut tree in our yard.

'Each time you come back you learn more,' Christina says. 'More self-awareness. To fight PTSD, you have to look deep into yourself.'

Journal entry. Ward 17, Melbourne. Sept 11, 2018: I've been thinking about the years I've lost because of PTSD. It doesn't frustrate me per se. I've sort of accepted it because I know now – from this admission – what I need to do.

A few days before my discharge, Cath does her group session on meaning and values again. There are a bunch of new patients in the ward. My four remaining values are:

Family-oriented
- *Family means everything to me.*
- *For so long I haven't been fully present for them. I want to change this so much.*

Love
- *Mary. Patrick. Belle. Harry.*
- *They love me. I love them. But I'm not showing my love enough.*

Honesty
- *Without honesty there can be no trust.*
- *I'm happy with my honesty. But being at Ward 17 (again) shows I sometimes need to be more honest with myself about how I'm travelling.*

Empathy
- *Putting yourself in someone else's shoes.*
- *Listening. Caring.*

It's not enough to say Mary, Patrick, Belle and Harry are the most important thing in the world. I need to show it. That means making self-care my top priority. Do that and they get the best of me. Without realising it, I've also begun the process of reshaping my identity to one that doesn't need the validation of being a successful journalist. It's anchored instead around being a good partner and father.

17

Wobbly

I'm relaxed and optimistic as the plane descends over Tasmania's green paddocks and water-logged rivers. Mary, on the other hand, is stressed, though I don't know it yet. Has this admission really been life changing, as I said on the phone from Ward 17? Mary picks me up from the airport and we have lunch in Launceston before she drives to Hobart for a two-day conference on trauma and the refugee community.

Mary has been counselling refugees for nearly two years. Her clients come from countries including Afghanistan, Ethiopia, Eritrea, South Sudan and Libya. Mary often talks about the battle they face trying to rebuild their shattered lives in Launceston. Many in this community of around 2000 speak poor English and have little chance of getting professional help for the complex trauma they carry. GPs and psychologists don't like working with interpreters. The refugees contend with poor job prospects, racism and a system that seems to say: well, you're out of the warzone, get on with it.

While Mary doesn't share confidential information, I know she listens to gut-wrenching stories every day. She fights for her clients against a cruel federal government that makes their lives harder or a legal system that doesn't always understand why trauma has put them in the dock. She believes the basic rights of her clients as people must be met for them to benefit from her counselling: broken windows and door locks must be fixed for her rape survivors, visas secured for parents still in overseas refugee camps. Mary's boss calls her a ferocious advocate for her clients, which makes me proud of her (again). I later get the words 'Ferocious Advocacy' tattooed on the inside of my left bicep.

Over lunch I give Mary earrings I bought for her birthday and talk about what I learned in Ward 17. She is quiet; she's heard variations of this story before. She is also disappointed I didn't return a day earlier so we could spend time together before she went to Hobart.

Patrick, Belle and Harry give me big hugs when they get home from school. Patrick is in grade 12 and plans to study Fine Arts at the University of Tasmania campus in Launceston but wants to take a gap year first. Belle brings me up to speed on news about our dog, four cats, multiple chickens, two rabbits and three sheep. Harry and I talk about the new songs he can play on his Fender Jaguar electric guitar. I cook fried rice for dinner.

I sleep well, only to wake around dawn when the dog barks. The kids go to school. I'm tired but make it to a mid-morning Bikram Yoga class, which invigorates me, and later do a walk. Something making a difference already is my new mantra: *Set your intention*. OT Michelle drummed the words into us at Ward 17: set your intention to understand your PTSD, she had said. For me, it's become *set your intention* to meditate, *set your intention* to go to Bikram. Those three words will soon be tattooed on the inside of my right bicep.

Harry comes to my study after school, curious about the patients in Ward 17. All good people, I say, trying to make their way in life. He asks if I want to watch a movie. You bet. Later I take Belle to a party in Launceston. I'm exhausted by bedtime. I miss not having Mary to cuddle.

I'm anxious the next morning. It's the pace of home life. Housework needs doing and the kids aren't helping. I want things tidy before Mary gets home. I have a good walk and do 60 sit-ups in the living room. I meditate in the radiant warmth of the wood-fired heater, rain on the roof slows my breathing. By early afternoon, my anxiety has faded. Then Mary arrives, stressed and hypervigilant.

'I feel awful saying this, but I'm worried how long your stability will last,' she says.

I've had three admissions to a psych ward in two years. Mary's anxiety is understandable. Just as Maryam told me there would be no quick fix, no aha moment in my own recovery, it's the same for Mary.

'You must be honest with me. This is the reality of PTSD,' I reply.

What neither of us realises is that this fear and anxiety has gotten locked in Mary's body. Years of worrying about me, making sure the kids are safe, ready to grab them and bolt if necessary.

The next morning, Saturday, Mary and I drive Harry to his guitar lesson in Launceston. While waiting, we have our first proper chat since my discharge. I tell Mary how much I love her. I describe the warm feelings in my stomach for her. It was in Ward 17 that I realised how wrong I was to justify visiting sex workers by saying it was only physical, that it meant nothing, I say.

'I've realised fully, for the first time, how destructive that was to our marriage. I am so sorry.'

Being a man, and stupid, I think it's fine to veer from my infidelity to love-making with my partner, and suggest we try having sex every weekend.

I think we've had a great conversation, but Mary hadn't been expecting this. The next morning, she is deeply stressed about how I'll cope with home life over the coming weeks and months. And it's too soon for sex, she says. She'd woken during the night, thinking: *I can't do this. I'm not ready.*

'Before we can begin having sex, I need to heal,' she says gently.

I understand, I reply. I really *did*. I didn't feel rejected. I was ashamed of my behaviour, what I'd done to Mary. What I didn't realise was that getting Mary to trust me again would be one thing, releasing the trauma locked in her body far more complex.

Mary also says no to renewing our marriage vows. She said yes when I raised it in Ward 17 the previous week but has changed her mind. She needs to feel safe, and not just in the bedroom. She wants to sort out everything from our finances to decluttering the house and yard.

I try to meditate in bed that afternoon, but I'm too anxious and itch all over.

Mary comes in, says she knows she is pushing me.

'You are,' I reply. 'But we need this honesty. Our relationship won't heal without it. And let's face it, I'm the cause of all the problems.'

I have only a few drinks that evening but feel like getting hammered.

Mary wakes up during the night again and sits in the living room. She's been thinking about me seeing sex workers before I had PTSD.

'I've been wondering if you were addicted to sex,' Mary says the next morning.

'I know I had a high sex-drive, I'm just not sure what addiction means in this context,' I reply.

None of my Ward 17 treating team used addiction to describe my sexual behaviour. But that evening it hits me, what a disgusting person I am. I wake the next day feeling depressed and worthless. Mary is in the kitchen about to go to work.

'I don't deserve you and never have,' I say, staring at the floor. I want to hurt myself. Cutting comes to mind. 'You deserve so much better than me.'

'I know how much you respect women and want to fight for women,' Mary says, leaving the inevitable question hanging in the air – how do I reconcile what I did to her with who I think I am or want to be?

Silence descends between us. I'm still staring at the floor.

'I don't know if I can cope with this,' Mary says.

'I'm going back to bed,' is all I can muster.

'Do you need to go back to Ward 17?'

I've been home for seven days.

—

The Guardian's chief culture writer Charlotte Higgins says patriarchy is the multilayered oppression of women. It operates through inequalities at home, work, the legal system and the state. Powerful cultural norms, education and religion uphold the patriarchy so that it seems natural or inevitable, or, in a liberal context, is obscured by piecemeal advances in gender equality, Higgins writes. Because patriarchy 'offers the idea of a structure of power relations rather than a series of specific sexist acts, it accommodates the idea that not all men enthusiastically uphold it or benefit equally from it'.

I think patriarchy partly explains why I never felt guilt or shame over visiting sex workers while married to Mary. As a man, part of me felt entitled to the physical pleasure. When we met in Hong Kong in 1995, I had the stable job, but Mary was the one hitting home runs with her stories. Nevertheless, we moved to Singapore two years later for my work. There was no real discussion; it was just taken for granted.

Yet I saw myself as 100 per cent progressive on gender issues, always have. I've done the cooking at home for years and pitch in to help with cleaning and washing.

My reaction to Mary's unexpected pregnancy in 2006 reeked of patriarchy. About five minutes after I told Dr Maryam during my first admission that I wanted to write to Namir and Saeed, she asked if I'd heard of Italian journalist Oriana Fallaci and her book, *Letter to a Child Never Born*.

I hadn't.

'You haven't heard of her! Surely you have, you're a journalist!' Maryam said.

I scratched my head, racked my brain, but Oriana Fallaci didn't ring a bell.

Born in 1929, Fallaci earned fame for long and revealing interviews with leaders such as Indira Gandhi, Yasser Arafat, Henry Kissinger, Deng Xiaoping, Ayatollah Khomeini and Muammar Gaddafi. She also wrote several books, including *Letter to a Child Never Born*. Published in 1975, the book recounts the dialogue Fallaci had with her unborn child following an unwanted pregnancy until she miscarried three months later. The book was translated into dozens of languages, including Persian, which was how Maryam read it.

Maryam brought up Fallaci because we had talked on several occasions about my reaction to Mary's unexpected pregnancy. How could I have been so cold and calculating? I'd said to Maryam. I ruminated over this in Ward 17. Was that why Mary miscarried, the stress and anguish I caused her? I hated myself.

Back home in late September 2016 after my first admission, I wrote Mary a 1400-word letter over a couple of days. In it, I explained how I got the idea from my conversation with Maryam about Oriana Fallaci. I found Mary in her study and asked if I could read her something. I held two printed pages, my hands shaking slightly. Mary was puzzled until I began:

'A Letter to my Sweet Wife and the Child Who Was Never Born.'

When you told me you were pregnant back in early 2006, I was stunned . . .

Did my heartless reaction cause you to have a miscarriage that night, sweet baby? I feel that in some way I must have been responsible. The timing could not have been a coincidence. I know this will cause you pain, to have to relive this again. But my reaction was inexcusable and inhuman. How could I be so heartless? I am ashamed.

I know how much you grieved for our lost child, babe. I would be lying if I said I too grieved. I don't think I did. But I thought a lot about how much I hurt you while I was in Ward 17.

One day in Ward 17, I also thought about our lost child.

Would you have been a boy or a girl? It would not have mattered of course. What would you be like now? I'm sure we would have marvelled at our youngest child . . . Going through PTSD has given me a new awareness of the importance of family and just how much my family loves me unconditionally. I return that love unconditionally, although I haven't always shown it in recent years.

If I could have any moment over again in my life, babe, it would be that moment when you first told me you were pregnant.

That letter meant a lot to Mary. I couldn't write to Namir and Saeed before I'd written to you, I told Mary. I felt emotion in my body, but I didn't really show any. What was wrong with me? Mary still grieves for our lost child. Did I? I wasn't sure what grieving meant.

When Jo Fidgen from the BBC asked me a few months later on the *Outlook* program if I'd written any letters to Mary, I told her she must be looking through a crystal ball. Mary said she would have been fine for me to talk about the letter on air, but I wasn't ready for that sort of disclosure.

Mary grieves the loss of another child who died in Jakarta that night in 2006. His name was Oki and he had stage four bone cancer.

Mary had set up a foundation in 2003 with an Indonesian paediatrician to raise money for impoverished parents who couldn't afford chemotherapy for their terminally ill children. She raised money from expatriates in Jakarta, foreign schools and companies, as well as wealthy Indonesians. The funds paid for X-rays, blood tests and CT scans, and chemotherapy. Mary allocated a child to a sponsor and provided updates through printed short stories and photos. Sponsors saw how (all) their money was spent. When an oncologist called Dr Edi Setiawan Tehuteru, whom Mary had met, was tasked with setting up Indonesia's first children's cancer ward at the Kanker Dharmais Hospital in Jakarta, he sought help from what Mary called her seat-of-the-pants operation. Government funding was available, but many parents were barely literate or didn't have the right documents. Others didn't understand the nightmarish paper-work. Besides, there often wasn't time if their children needed urgent treatment.

By the time families reached hospital, the cancer was usually critical, and the bread-earner had left or lost his or her job to bring the family to Jakarta. Most families had travelled from far-flung parts of the world's largest archipelago. Siblings had been pulled out of school. Families had sold everything, borrowed from loan sharks. Indonesia was the country worst hit by the Asian finan-cial crisis in the late 1990s.

Most children eventually died because their cancer was late stage. But Dr Edi never gave up and Mary kept raising money, which included support for children with leukaemia. The charity paid debts and, when a child died, funeral expenses. In some cases, it allowed a child to die at home with dignity, as well as help families get back on their feet. Mary promised herself that she'd be there each time a child died in the cancer ward.

Mary had been called that night to the hospital because Oki, eleven, was dying. She wanted to be with Oki and his parents but couldn't because she was losing our child. Oki's mother was heavily pregnant and later named her baby girl Rhamat Mary.

I never appreciated what Mary did until volunteers who had helped Mary gave her a farewell party before we left Indonesia. I didn't see the point in Mary spending so much time on the charity if she wasn't getting paid and it was taking her away from our kids. At the party – the volunteers renamed the charity Mary's Cancer Kiddies – I grasped the enormity of what she had done. Years later, Mary said she believed a part of me wanted to avoid the sadness of dying children and suffering parents, especially because

I spoke Indonesian. She was half-right. In 2021, Mary's Cancer Kiddies became a registered foundation and was renamed Yayasan Mari Cintai Kanak-Kanak (Let's Love the Children Foundation). Proud her humble operation was thriving, Mary, who hates the spotlight, was nevertheless relieved her name had been removed.

—

On that day at home when I'm too ashamed to look Mary in the eye, a week after my latest discharge from Ward 17, I finally see through the bullshit I've spun all these years. I talk about being betrayed by Reuters ad nauseam. What about my betrayal of Mary? What a hypocrite. Rebuilding trust with Mary will take time. Right now, I can set my intention to get my self-care routine on track. I can do that for Mary and my family. Then they get the best of me. That is one way I can atone.

Journal entry. Evandale, Tasmania. Sept 20, 2018: It's been a massive change coming home, especially given the issues Mary and I have been addressing. This has generated a lot of emotion, which is why it's so important to have my self-care routine nailed down.

The next day I exercise early. I meditate and even do Tai Chi. I decide to get off social media. I've been posting regularly about my journey and mental health issues in general. I'm not an avid user, but it's a distraction. My mood improves.

I know I'm feeling good when I get my latest tattoo and the needle hurts. Before my third Ward 17 admission, I craved the pain. Then, the needle was a drug, nearly as important as the narrative on my skin. Mary loves the tattoo – *PTSD 'Not a Life Sentence'* across the inside of my left forearm.

It's nearly six weeks since my discharge. My self-care regime is going well. Mary drove a long discussion on our finances and we've got a proper budget in place.

A couple of days later I fly to Sydney to give a speech at the annual dinner of an Australian company that makes armoured vehicles for special forces around the world. I went to university with its managing director, Mick Halloran. I speak for 45 minutes about my career, PTSD, Ward 17 admissions and good mental health in the workplace.

I get an Uber to a friend's place, replaying the evening in my mind. The meaning I got from it. I check my phone, which I've barely looked at all night. DZ has messaged me.

The man who raped DZ has been exonerated, again. DZ thought he'd be fired. I did too.

DZ: *My complaints were not upheld.*

DZ: *I am doing ok.*

DZ: *I will talk to you sometime next week, when things are more settled.*

Me: *I am so sorry to hear that. I can't believe it. I'm truly shocked for you. I'm here whenever you want to talk, next week or earlier. Just let me know.*

I'm stunned. How was this possible? The person who investigated DZ's complaint is a high-profile lawyer who later becomes a judge.

The following week I fall into a deep depression. After much speculation inside Reuters, the company says a series of job losses will be announced over the coming months as part of a major restructuring called Newsroom of the Future. The cuts will coincide with an inaugural week-long campaign on mental health and switching off from the 24/7 news cycle, that I've organised for mid-November. My boss says the campaign, called Mental Health Week, will have to be postponed. Colleagues might see it as a box-ticking exercise to mollify staff. I agree and don't want people thinking that. I draft the following note, which goes to the company's comms department in New York for approval.

Dear Colleagues – In light of the announcement on job losses, we've decided to postpone mental health week until sometime in the first half of 2019. Some might think this is the perfect time to hold mental health week given the distress and uncertainty over job losses. My concern is that mental health week will be seen as a token attempt to deal with these totally understandable emotions. Or worse, a pre-meditated move to try to placate staff. Neither would be true. I want mental health week to be the signature event we hold each year to focus on the wellbeing of our people. That means delaying until the time is right.

Someone cuts all references to job losses. I fight the revisions for nearly two weeks, to no avail, and the note circulates just before Mental Health Week is supposed to begin. A senior colleague emails me, saying redundancies won't be good for anyone's mental health.

I think about resigning. I worry that my credibility with staff is in tatters. I've got little to show for a year's work. A recent proposal I'd made to create a mental health team to support Reuters journalists had been rejected with virtually no discussion. Such a team could have helped me create transparent policies on stress, burnout, mental illness, trauma, substance abuse, sexual harassment and bullying, I'd written. Staff would have felt more comfortable talking to their manager and/or HR about these issues if clear guidelines existed, I'd argued.

My self-care routine goes out the window. The nightmares return. I start drinking and withdraw from Mary. One day after a misunderstanding over something that seemed trivial, Mary leaves the house upset, won't talk to me. After a while, I drive around Evandale trying to find her. I panic. Mary is at the South Esk River, the one place I don't look.

'I wonder if your PTSD is too big for us,' Mary says.

Fear grips my insides. Is this the end? But Mary is giving voice to what's been in my head, too. She's just had the courage to say it.

Do I need to move out? I ask Mary. No, she says, but we need to be clearer in our communication with each other.

'I don't mean this as a criticism, but it's so hard living with someone with PTSD,' she says.

I initially think: *What Mary means is what Reuters did to me.* But what I'd done, what I keep doing, is giving myself a get-out-of-jail-free card called Reuters. By blaming the organisation for everything, I don't have to take responsibility for anything. I'm looking outwards. Not inwards. One evening Mary said to me: 'I look at you and all I see is Reuters.' I'm not reflecting on my behaviour over many years and what I need to do to heal my relationship with Mary.

A few days later, my psychologist Wendy Gall tells me it's normal for strains to emerge in a relationship that has been through crisis after crisis. It shows things are getting back to normal. You might be less tolerant with each other, Wendy says. Issues suppressed for a long time, especially for Mary, are being addressed. Mary is calling a spade a spade.

That night Mary and I walk down to our local pub, the Prince of Wales. It's a typical Tasmanian rural pub, deer head with antlers mounted on the wall, men in flannelette shirts and riding boots at the bar. Wendy's comments help us put things in perspective. Now it's my turn to be honest.

I need to quit Reuters, I tell Mary. I don't want to abandon my colleagues, but the stress is too much. I need more control over my life. Mary is a bit surprised but understands. We talk options and agree not to make hasty decisions. It might take six to twelve months to devise an alternative career plan. Preparing for the future will help you deal with these frustrations, Mary replies.

We talk about our life together, the kids, our travels, the stories we covered, friends. We express gratitude for what we have.

Luckily I'm about to take two months long-service leave. It's early December and the weather is warming up. One day I take Belle out for lunch. Belle recently turned eighteen and has finished grade 11. She got a tattoo of an Indonesian gecko, a *chi chak*, across her left shoulder blade for her birthday. Belle has had a good year, settling into a new public school, getting great marks in art. She is considering becoming a vet nurse. Belle doesn't just connect with animals; she can sense when they are unwell. And her perceptiveness extends to people. If I'm only slightly off kilter, Belle will deliberately look at me and ask: 'How are you?'

After Belle and I chat for a bit, I take her hand and tell her there is something I need to say. Belle tenses, her eyes locked on mine.

'Sweetie, I am so sorry for the way I spoke to you all those years ago when you lit matches in your room,' I say.

Belle's face dissolves, tears roll down her cheeks.

'I was horrible. Rather than try to understand what was going on, I shouted at you. PTSD did that. It wasn't your father. I love you so much and am so sorry for hurting you. And I'm so sorry for taking so long to apologise.'

I ask Belle to forgive me, which she does, then she gives me a warm hug.

—

It's been two and a half months since my discharge. I'm feeling good; walking, meditating, and writing daily, eating well. In bed I want to be naked with my brave and beautiful partner. Mary murmurs with pleasure when I put my hand up her nightshirt and rub her back but still freezes if I move to her thigh. I think she is traumatised. Sex with me went from something special, passionate, to something she hated. Those memories have been burned into her body. There was no 'equality in our intimacy', Mary says. 'Be patient with me.'

I *really* get it. The extent of what I've done is dawning on me. It might take a long time for Mary to heal.

On New Year's Eve 2018, Mary and I have dinner at the Prince of Wales.

'This recovery is real,' I say.

'I prefer the word healing,' Mary says.

My mind searches for a better word.

'I am managing this. I am managing my PTSD.'

'You are more self-aware of when you need to rest or exercise,' says Mary.

'I might still sleep in the afternoon, but it's different to before. Then, I was exhausted or depressed. Now it's about having a rest. It's enjoyable.'

Mary has carved out a new career she loves. Patrick is taking a gap year. Belle is going into grade 12 and Harry grade 11. And I've got a plan, start preparing a future away from Reuters that will revolve around writing, public speaking, and workplace mental health consulting.

Mary and I walk home and sit on a bench seat to watch the sky turn red as the sun drifts towards the Western Tiers. The chooks amble down to their wooden coop. Mas Biru, Mary's favourite cat, sits next to her.

Life is good.

I get up early on New Year's Day, full of optimism. Strips of sunlight angle across the brown paddocks as I stretch my leg muscles. The South Esk River is low enough to walk across. Birdsong fills the air. It's going to be warm. I glide around Evandale's deserted streets, rock music pumping through my headphones. I write while waiting for Mary to wake. We plan to garden before it gets too hot.

Around late morning Mary and I are out the front when I realise I forgot to close the backyard gate. Shit, has Lois gotten out? Our turbo-charged labrador will go for the chickens. This happened before and there were casualties. I sprint to where I think the chooks might be.

A second later, squawking chickens fly in all directions. The golden-coloured lab has Belle's favourite chook, a white Silky called Marge, in her jaws. I scream at Lois, who looks at me, poised for action. Lois loves being chased but knows I'm not playing. She drops Marge and takes off. I run after Lois through hedges and garden beds and around the shed. I slip over a couple of times, getting angrier.

After a few minutes, Belle grabs Lois when she slows to snatch another chook. I get Lois by the scruff of the neck, wanting to strangle this dog cowering at my feet. My heart pounds. I've screamed myself hoarse. Mary comes over and leads Lois away. I stand up, panting, and kick wildly at dry grass and weeds. Calm down, Mary says, or words to that effect.

'You don't understand what this does to my brain,' I shout at Mary, two or three times.

Mary puts Lois in the living room and sits with me on the step outside. I'm hyperventilating.

'What can you do to bring yourself down?' Mary asks.

'Things had been going so well,' I say, gulping in air.

'This is fine, it just shows that even after many good weeks you can still be affected,' Mary replies.

I itch all over, between my fingers, up my forearms to my face. Sweat drips off me. My head starts to throb. I'm dizzy.

One question turns over in my head, on a loop: *What just happened to my brain?*

I have a shower, take Panadol, and ask Mary to lie with me in bed. Two years ago, I would have left the room and said nothing, so this is progress. When I get up, I still have a headache. I wolf down a loaf of banana bread Belle has cooked for me. Baking trays fall from the top cupboard as Belle puts things away. She cringes. I hear a barely audible 'sorry'.

'It's okay, sweetie, I saw it happening.'

Exhaustion slams me. I sleep more and still have the headache. I take some of Mary's migraine medication, but it doesn't work. My anger was scary. Then there is shame. Mary and Belle shouldn't have seen me like that.

Mary comes in and says it's okay, they're just chooks and a dog. I sleep for a bit, get up. I watch TV, make Mary a salad. By 7 pm I'm done. I go to bed, telling Mary why. She understands. I wait for depression to drop. I take two Valium, then another one twenty minutes later which eventually knocks me out. My body needs two days to recover.

What happened to my brain?

*

I never tried to get my head around the brain stuff during three admissions to Ward 17. Too much science. This deprived me of an understanding of the emotional, unconscious part of the brain, also known as the limbic system.

Lois changes that.

I open a book by renowned American clinician Babette Rothschild called *The Body Remembers: The Psychophysiology of Trauma and Trauma Treatment*, published in 2000. Understanding how the brain and body process and *perpetuate* (my emphasis) traumatic events is key to recovery, Rothschild writes.

She explains that the limbic system regulates survival behaviour and emotional expression, thus mediating arousal levels. It's the limbic system's relationship with the autonomic nervous system (ANS) that matters most for someone with PTSD. (The ANS is a sub-branch of the central nervous system.)

The limbic system sends signals to the ANS to either prepare the body for action or to let it rest. The ANS has two branches: the sympathetic nervous system (SNS), which is for action, and the parasympathetic nervous system (PNS), which is for rest. If someone is confronted with a threat, the amygdala, the brain's lightning-fast but unsophisticated guard dog, activates the SNS and pumps hormones such as adrenaline into the body to mobilise for fight or flight. If death is imminent or escape impossible, the limbic system can activate the PNS instead, causing the body to freeze or go into a state of tonic immobility. These responses are instantaneous survival actions. The SNS and PNS usually work in balance: when one rises, the other suppresses and vice versa.

PTSD is characterised, in part, by chronic ANS hyper-arousal, adds Rothschild. This helps explain why people with PTSD are so vulnerable to stress. The system is always stressed.

When SNS arousal is constantly high, adding new stress pushes it higher, and it doesn't take much to feel overwhelmed. That's why people with PTSD can't handle daily stress like others or like they used to.

The body doesn't return to equilibrium for people with PTSD, writes Bessel van der Kolk in *The Body Keeps the Score*. Fight, flight and freeze signals keep going off after the danger has passed and the continued secretion of hormones is expressed as agitation, panic, anxiety and anger.

This makes sense, but why would a bloody dog chasing chickens trigger me so badly? There was no danger to me or a loved one.

When I next see Wendy, she says yes, my amygdala went into fight mode. Lois was the trigger. I didn't consciously choose to chase her. My brain did. It assessed the situation in a split second: Lois likely to kill chickens, bloodied carcasses, daughter upset. Wendy says memories from somewhere like Iraq might have also been aroused in my body by the noise in the yard, the chase, Mary, Belle and myself shouting.

Rothschild writes that people with PTSD can't make sense of their symptoms in the context of the events they've endured. These traumatic experiences 'free-float in time without an end or place in history'. The thing to understand is that PTSD can make it hard to recognise the present as being different from the past. Okay, I could see I wasn't in Baghdad, but my body might have thought otherwise when I ran after Lois. To use Rothschild's words, my nervous system might have been fooled into thinking something from the past was being repeated. Adds van der Kolk: '[People with PTSD] have no idea why they respond to some minor irritation as if they were about to be annihilated . . . The challenge is not so much learning to accept the terrible things that have happened but learning how to gain mastery over one's internal sensations and emotions. Sensing, naming, and identifying what is going on inside is the first step to recovery.'

Wendy says I can't control my sensory environment to the point where I risk nothing happening. I need to train myself so that after a moment, I can bring myself under control.

'When you know why something happens, it takes away some of the mystery, the uncertainty,' she says. 'It also helps that you are telling yourself, *This is life*. You cannot shut yourself off and expect your family to do the same.'

Once I understand how the autonomic nervous system works, I get curious. When I get stressed, I say to myself: Okay, what caused that? Why did I startle? Or why didn't I startle when I normally would have? Or what do I need to do to activate my PNS?

Suddenly, my world changes.

Harry and I go to Sydney to see American rock band Greta Van Fleet play at the Enmore Theatre at the end of January. I don't need headphones on the crowded streets. I don't get anxious trying to find taxis. The crowds at Darling Harbour where we stay don't bother me. I've been exercising, doing Bikram Yoga, eating well in the past couple of weeks, so that has helped.

A few days later, back home, Lois gets out again. This time Harry raises the alarm and rushes inside to tell me. Belle is also there. They look at me aghast, like I'll blow a fuse, and are amazed when I barely react.

It's just a dog and chickens.

18

What is wrong with these people?

L oss of control is at the heart of PTSD.

'No one develops PTSD who was in control of the circumstances: able to stop the car or the tsunami, not be in the wrong place at the wrong time, avoid the perpetrator and so on,' writes Babette Rothschild. PTSD's symptoms also appear beyond the sufferer's control. Therefore, it makes sense for therapists to help clients try to reclaim and increase control over their body, mind, therapy and life, Rothschild says in *The Body Remembers Volume 2: Revolutionizing Trauma Treatment*.

Those words jumped off the page when I read them about a week after chasing Lois around the yard. For so long I had control over my life. Did well at school, got a university degree. Never bullied, never had my heart broken, married a wonderful woman. Financial stability. No major health issues until PTSD.

From the moment I joined Reuters as a young reporter in Jakarta in 1993 my bosses supported me, gave me opportunities and responsibility. Even as my PTSD symptoms mounted and my family suffered, I was getting the highest performance rating each year. This helped me deny the reality of my mental state. How can there be anything wrong when I'm a top performer? With so much of my identity tied up in my career, I still felt, weirdly perhaps, in control of my life. Reuters destroyed that when it made me feel like damaged goods and tried to force me out of the company.

Mary and I are discussing Rothschild's latest book over breakfast one Saturday morning. I show Mary the passages I've highlighted about control. Mary is familiar with Rothschild's books. They helped her understand that some of her refugee clients make little progress in therapy because they have no control over their lives: language barriers; no work; lack of access to transport; confusing government bureaucracy; racism; family members stuck in warzones or refugee camps. They have no bandwidth for therapy.

'That is powerlessness,' Mary says, referring to her clients. 'And I think that the loss of control for men, for someone like you, equates to powerlessness.'

I put my cup of tea on the table and sit back in my chair. I've never described myself as powerless in roughly 250,000 words of journal entries up to this moment. But that is exactly what Reuters did after I was diagnosed with PTSD. Made me feel powerless. And it was deeply shaming because it all unfolded in front of my family, and I couldn't do anything about it.

'Powerlessness leads to shame which leads to anger,' I reply to Mary, who nods.

I suddenly understand how my anger at Reuters connects – the moral injury, the betrayal, the powerlessness, and the shame. It dawns on me that this trauma is as much about the loss of control of my life story as anything. I need to regain control of my narrative. Until I do, I'll never heal.

I thought I'd made a breakthrough six months ago in Ward 17. I was wrong. The wound is too deep. One day I'm reading *The Choice* by Edith Eger, who was a Hungarian teenager when the Nazis sent her and her family to the Auschwitz death camp in 1944. Her parents were killed in gas chambers. Eger and her sister survived until the war ended. Eger became a well-known psychologist in the United States and published her book at 90.

She never harboured fantasies of revenge.

How is that possible? I feel pathetic, locked in chains with an organisation that gave me an extraordinary and well-paid career. Then again, I gave them everything too.

Journal entry. Evandale, Tasmania. Jan 6, 2019: I WILL NEVER ACCEPT WHAT WAS DONE TO ME IN 2016. EVER. Who knew what and when? Who was determining my fate? Who knew in advance about the Oct 17 email? Who was consulted?

I talk to Mary about Eger's book, playing down the fact I'm obsessing (again) about Reuters, saying I can't forgive or let go. Mary says it might take time. 'I'd be surprised if you'd forgiven Reuters. Would that be real?' she asks.

Something that sticks in my head from Eger's book is the word accountability.

'Nothing is gained if we close our eyes to wrong, if we give someone a pass, if we dismiss accountability,' she writes. 'But as my fellow survivors taught me, you can live to avenge the past, or you can live to enrich the present.'

How does one seek accountability without it seeming like payback? I'm treading a fine line, thinking vengeful thoughts while wanting to create policies at Reuters that ensure no one gets treated like myself, DZ and other colleagues. Will telling my story set me free?

I also decide to throw the notion of managing my PTSD out the window. It's an arm's-length concept. In *Trauma and Recovery*, Judith Herman says the guiding principle of recovery is to restore power and control to the survivor. 'Control my PTSD' becomes my new mantra. But I misunderstand experts such as Rothschild and Herman, interpreting control as needing to be total, which wasn't what they meant.

Because I'm still on long-service leave, my mental state is good. I declutter my study, hang a full-sized Iraqi sword from Najaf on the wall in its sand-coloured metal scabbard. My Iraqi staff showered me with gifts when I left Baghdad at the end of 2008: the sword, a smaller curved traditional knife, paintings, a chess set, even presents for Mary. When we moved to Australia in early 2013, a worried shipping company official called to say customs had held up my container because I hadn't declared a weapon. I was puzzled, then remembered the sword. I also get the Iraqi national flag signed by my staff mounted and hung on the wall.

Mary is taking annual leave. We discuss what we've learnt about trauma, our work, each other.

'While it's been tough, your journey has enriched us both,' Mary says.

I'm in awe of Mary's determination to stick it out with me. I know it's about love and keeping our family together, but is this a woman thing too? Is it in their wiring because they are nurturers? Do men have that devotion to something greater than themselves when the chips are down?

Because I'm open about my mental health issues, people share their stories. One common theme is that if a woman has a mental illness, her male partner often gets itchy feet. When the shoe is on the other foot, the woman stays. A woman cutting my hair in Launceston lowered her voice as she told me how hard it was at home because of her husband's bipolar disorder. 'None of my co-workers know,' she said. I know a young woman whose husband left when she checked herself into a psych ward to treat her depression and anxiety. The husband of another woman who developed PTSD from childhood sexual abuse moved out, leaving her with their three young children. A man has never approached me after my public talks to seek advice about his partner. Women do it all the time, during the event and later. I suspect men also run because mental illness can be a handbrake on sex.

One day Mary says clearly for the first time that fear is stopping her from making love with me. Trauma is locked in her body.

I tell Wendy Gall that what I did to Mary was the same as violating her, forcing her to do something against her will. But I'm still obsessing outwards, at my frustration with Reuters. The reminders, the triggers, every time I get an email. It's hard to move forward when there is no accountability, apology or even acknowledgement, Wendy says. I'm not sure if she does this deliberately – but Wendy cites a cheating husband. I shift uncomfortably in my chair. 'If he blames his wife – you're not giving me what I want – why should she stay? If he is deeply remorseful, you can work with that.'

My attempt to control my PTSD takes a hit a few weeks later, when, back at work in February after long-service leave, I'm told key elements of my proposed mental health strategy for 2019 are non-starters, and that my role should be made part-time. Though Reuters will still pay me a full wage. My job won't occupy all my time this year, which might frustrate me, hurt my recovery. I'm told, gently, to think about opportunities outside Reuters such as professional study or an attachment with the Dart Center for Journalism and Trauma in New York.

My mind freezes for a couple of days. I want to quit but Mary and Jeremy persuade me to stay, saying it's too soon and that I should try to leave on my own terms.

A few months later – I've ignored the part-time thing – the legal department wants to gut a mobile-friendly website on mental health for Reuters journalists which I've spent eighteen months creating. Something about liability. Then I'm blocked from arranging a meeting with the news leadership when I'll be in London, New York and Washington in October.

I'm done, I tell Mary and one or two close colleagues. I'll do my overseas trip because Mental Health Week has been rescheduled for early October and a lot of work has gone into organising it with the peer network. I also want to train more managers on how to look after the mental health of their staff and hold separate forums for anyone on dealing with stress. Then I'll give my resignation to the bosses in New York.

I happen to be in Sydney when my efforts to meet the news leadership are scuttled. The Australia bureau chief has asked me to brief Kim Williams, chairman of the Thomson Reuters Founders Share Company, about my work. Kim is a well-known Australian who has run numerous media, arts and entertainment businesses including News Ltd, now News Corp Australia. The Founders Share Company has a duty to ensure the Reuters Trust Principles of integrity, independence and freedom from bias are maintained. These principles, drawn up in 1941 during World

War Two, are the cornerstone of Reuters journalism. They are why surveys show the company is one of the most trusted news organisations in the world.

Kim is visiting the Sydney bureau for the day.

I keep it professional, giving a presentation on the mental health initiatives in place and others I'm working on. He's impressed with the website, called the Reuters Mental Health & Resilience Resource. Kim asks if I might be in London in early October to address the board of the Founders Share Company at its annual meeting. What a coincidence, I reply.

A meeting is set up for me to speak to a board filled with global business, media and human rights figures. I start planning a speech on the resistance to my work and the impact this is having on Reuters journalists. Mary and Jeremy talk me out of it, urging me to take the opportunity to win powerful allies instead.

About ten days before flying out, I go and see Steve Biddulph, a neighbour who is also one of the world's best-known psychotherapists. Steve wrote the best-selling books *Raising Boys, Raising Girls* and *The New Manhood*. I first met Steve and his wife Shaaron when one of our pet rabbits escaped its hutch and Mary and I went looking for it. Another time we dropped in Shaaron was nursing an orphaned pademelon in a cloth pouch around her neck. Their home was humble, and homely, and so were they.

Steve is tall and lanky at 68, with unruly hair. He has a gentle demeanour, though he can cut to the chase.

We have chatted often about trauma and mental health. He's taken a keen interest in the welfare of me and my family.

Steve – like Dr Maryam, Cath Taylor, Christina Sim, Wendy and of course Mary – has encouraged me to engage my emotions.

I'm not an easy convert. I rely on my prefrontal cortex, the part of the brain that controls executive function, to suppress what I don't want to feel.

'Control must be for life,' I tell Steve one morning in late September 2019 in his living room. 'Ease off and PTSD will move back in.' Without knowing it, I'm perched on the edge of a chair, pointing at the wall.

'Dean, are you aware of how you are sitting?' Steve says. 'Can you get more comfortable?'

Sheepishly I sit back in the armchair, the tension falling away. Steve doesn't labour the point, but he's trying to explain that I can choose how to breathe, hold my muscles. My stress is bad sometimes, but I can learn to *not* make it worse. To breathe through it, and of course to get help. Steve has a polar opposite view to the one I've formed on dealing with my PTSD, but today, I'm still ranting about Reuters and quickly forget what he said.

Steve must have expected this because he sends me an email a few days later. 'ALWAYS START WITH THE BODY,' he writes in capital letters. 'Just check out – are you comfortable, breathing, connected to gravity, what are the inner sensations? It's not about controlling things – it's that when you notice, you will automatically have more options and can change what you don't like. Control was a vital part of dealing with things in the past, and will be needed at times, but it's an emergency measure.'

—

In London, Mental Health Week goes well. Some of the bosses share how they manage stress and unplug. Colourful posters I had designed by a small marketing outfit in Tasmania are put up in newsrooms around the world. One says: *Vicarious Trauma is Real: There is no Shame in Asking for Support.* The peers have organised various activities: visits by assistance dogs in London and Washington, drawing lessons in Bangalore, and martial arts classes in Hong Kong. I write a blog called *Getting Control Of My PTSD, One Step At A Time* that is circulated within Reuters and posted on social media.

I present to the Founders Share Company board for 45 minutes on 10 October, World Mental Health Day. I show them the yet-to-be-launched Reuters Mental Health & Resilience Resource and explain why I think being a Reuters journalist today is tougher than at any time in history. I take questions, am thanked profusely, and Kim Williams invites me back to the board's next annual meeting. Sitting quietly in the room is the editor-in-chief.

In London, New York and Washington I run multiple sessions on dealing with stress and put dozens of managers through my training course that focuses on mental health literacy, spotting signs of distress and how to have a conversation with an employee. I designed the course based on research from Australia's Black Dog Institute.

At the same time, I'm still tussling with the legal department over final content for the website. They have watered down the information on sexual harassment, which I say is 'shockingly weak language and an insult to our female staff'. Since getting approval for the project nearly two years ago, I've wanted staff, stringers and family members to have information at their fingertips on stress, trauma and mental illness as well as self-care and how to get support. To my delight, my boss had agreed to make the resource public, meaning we could share our knowledge with the broader journalism community. Sam Harvey, chief psychiatrist at the Black Dog Institute, called the site an 'outstanding resource' for journalists after I showed him.

But the issue that dominates my trip, which comes up in almost every conversation, is the Newsroom of the Future demolition ball. Underway for nearly a year, the bosses want to overhaul the planning, coordination and editing of news among text, TV, pictures, data, graphics, digital, social media and online. It has taken on an almost Orwellian feel. The bosses talk of building 'smarter, simpler, more customer-focused and more journalist-friendly ways of working'.

When I ask colleagues from the peer network at their annual meeting in London what they think when I say 'Newsroom of the Future', they respond with: 'layoffs, job losses, chaos, jargon, corporate speak, removing layers of management only to create more layers, do more with less.' Journalists are overwhelmed with stress, bewildered and fearful, being asked to do the same amount of work (or more) with less staff. I get so concerned about one desking unit in London that I tell their boss in New York I suspect some are close to a mental breakdown. When I urge people to push back if they don't have the journalists for the demands coming their way, there is a near uniform response – 'I'm afraid I'll lose my job if I do that.' One multi prize–winning journalist says: 'I know it's irrational, but the thought has crossed my mind whether my job is safe.'

I'm furious at the suffering among colleagues but emboldened by their support for my work and buoyed after my presentation to the Founders Share Company. A plan forms in my head. I have meetings in New York over two days with a new global head of HR, the editor-in-chief and the president of Reuters. I decide to pitch for a two- to three-year mental health strategy with guiding principles, buy-in from the top and a proper budget.

Up to this point, strategy has never been debated and agreed with the leadership. I was informed six weeks into the role in early 2017 that my job description had been substantially revised. Gone was working with the external trauma support provider and the peer network because one or two bureaucrats were unnerved by what I might do and wanted to protect their turf. I submitted an 80-page blueprint for action in mid-2017 that called for a review of demands and expectations on staff because of the enormous stress on them – eighteen months before the Newsroom of the Future was launched. The report gathered dust. In April 2018 when I told my manager the leadership didn't trust me, he replied: 'There are questions of trust. It is trust but it isn't. The question is your passion. We have to make sure nothing goes haywire . . . We need to make sure people feel comfortable. Your passion makes people nervous.'

Around the time I was told this, I wanted to trial my manager training program in Beirut. I'd created the course based on a Black Dog Institute program that returned $10 for every $1 spent. It was an initiative endorsed by my bosses in New York. I chose Beirut because I knew people there, and felt it would make a good place to try the course given the stress colleagues were under from covering the war in Syria. HR had approved the course. Then a senior manager in London expressed concern.

When I called him, he said he understood I was passionate about staff mental health, and knew I believed this was vital for the company's future. There was a widespread view I was 'not wrong'. But the leadership was dealing with so many things, and then I throw in mental health and wellbeing, he said. The leadership had a 'tsunami of requirements'. We can't do it all, this person said. Secondly, the nature of what I was doing was unfamiliar and a 'little scary'. Probably because it's good but people were worried about change, he added. Thirdly, he cited his responsibility to bureaus. He was happy with me going to a bureau but what happened then? What if people needed time off because they discovered they were stressed? He'd need to reinforce those bureaus. I had to realise there could be repercussions for managers who had to 'pick up the pieces'. How do we deal with the consequences, he asked. There needed to be a plan in place.

I never went to Beirut but put nearly 100 managers through face-to-face courses in Singapore, New York, Washington and London in 2019.

The head of HR and the editor-in-chief seem amenable to my pitch after I talk about the stress staff are under. I tell the editor-in-chief I want to report to him to send a strong message to everyone that I have organisational authority and to ensure he knows what staff are going through. Staff contact me all the time about their stress and mental health issues, I say.

Then I see the president, who I've never met.

The president joined Reuters the previous December. I follow him into his spacious office on the 18th floor of Number 3 Times Square. He motions me to sit at a table with a few chairs around it. I'm drawn to something. The president is busying himself at his desk and doesn't notice my eyes widening in disbelief. I'm looking at work by the man who raped DZ, work that won him a major award. I do quick calculations: *Investigation wrapped up six weeks before president took over; doubt he knows about DZ; no one on this floor (HR/legal) or 19th (editorial) who knew about the investigation has said anything to him, like 'Hey, you might want to get rid of that'.*

Next thought, challenge him now or later? Decide to wait (coward) until I'm back in New York in December to speak at an international meeting of freelance journalists and hopefully my mental health strategy.

Last thought. What is wrong with these people?

—

Despite this unsettling moment, I arrive home relatively optimistic. The trip went better than expected, I tell Steve Biddulph in an email: 'I think I made major headway with the bosses, to the point where I think they will agree to me drawing up a mental health strategy . . . It would seem I still have a future with the organisation.'

I send the editor-in-chief a 1000-word email setting out what colleagues told me about their unrelenting stress and poor morale. I'd given him a taste when I met him, but it was time to spell it out in detail. I begin drafting the mental health strategy.

I also resume work with a new therapist, Dee Cooper, who is preparing me for a treatment called eye movement desensitisation and reprocessing (EMDR). Wendy Gall had suggested I try EMDR to deal with my anger. EMDR is one of the few evidence-based therapies approved to treat PTSD in Australia. I wasn't sure how it could help but I was ready to try anything. Dee is a clinical psychologist and the first fully accredited EMDR practitioner in Launceston.

Memories too intense for the brain to process define trauma, Dee has told me. EMDR aims to keep a survivor settled enough in the present moment to talk through an experience so it can be fully processed and committed to long-term memory instead of frozen in time. It can then be stored away, a bit like in the linen cupboard metaphor. The therapist does this by positioning their index finger in front of the client's eyes and asking them to follow the movement back and forth. The idea is to put just enough strain on the working memory, so the amygdala doesn't go bananas. This minimises the possibility of overwhelming emotion or dissociation. Dee took a case history during a couple of sessions before I went overseas and said she would focus on several specific elements of my anger and betrayal for EMDR when I got back.

Dee speaks with what sounds like a South African accent, though she was born in Zimbabwe. She has been a psychologist for 30 years. Like all my female clinicians, Dee doesn't hesitate to burst my bubble. Steve is right, she says. How can you control what happens inside your nervous system? Having pored over books on how the brain responds to trauma, I know the answer: YOU CAN'T. What I can do is try for more control over my response to a triggering event. But I can't control what my limbic system decides in a nano-second.

Dee continues to prepare me for EMDR, asking me to recall a moment in 2016 when I was truly frightened. I go back to being one brain-snap away from a *ledakan* (explosion). Dee digs into the circumstances. The Traumatic Stress Clinic in Sydney had just told me I couldn't get into their Skype program for five to six months. It had dawned on me how deeply my PTSD was affecting the kids. I couldn't take Harry to see his psychologist that day. I still hadn't submitted my proposal to train and mentor young reporters after more than two months of procrastinating. Telling Dee about these events, Reuters' indifference comes flooding back. I feel the fear in my body.

I go home drained from the session with Dee.

A few days later I have a blazing row with my boss, a colleague who has been suicidal seeks my help dealing with HR, and I stumble across recent work by the man who raped DZ. He is on a high-profile assignment. DZ is still off work. I slip into familiar patterns of depression and poor sleep. A colleague in the Middle East emails me, distressed about job losses in a region where she says almost every country is either at war or in revolution. A senior journalist in Africa says to me: 'You're like a microphone for everyone's concerns at the moment.'

Headaches combine with depression to flatten me. Mary has had a gutful. 'Enough is enough. You can't go on like this,' she says. 'You need to snap out of it. Your trip went well. Look at what you've achieved.'

I just don't know how to explain that I can't exist in a world where I breathe betrayal every day. Mary fears we won't be able to pay the mortgage on her wage alone if I resign. We might lose the house. She feels unsafe in the pit of her stomach.

I tell Dee I can't do EMDR. We haven't got to the finger waving stage. I take mental health leave, telling New York the root cause is the way Reuters treated me in 2016. I'm told to take as much time off as I need, but there is no acknowledgement the company might bear any responsibility. (In the interests of fairness, I want to make clear that all the people who caused my moral injury, turned a blind eye or failed to account for what happened have left Reuters. I hold no one in the present leadership responsible for that.)

The following morning, I see an email that has bounced around the peer network overnight. One peer from a far-flung part of the world is so aggrieved with management they sought advice from the 60-member group. Someone copied me in, suggesting I could help. I intervene aggressively, which leads to a testy email exchange with the same senior manager based in London who tells me to give the leadership credit instead of 'immediately jumping in and accusing us of neglect and dereliction of duty'. That day I hear that the leadership and dozens of other senior staff have just met in Canada to discuss the Newsroom of the Future. I wasn't told, let alone invited.

I ask the only person in a senior management position whom I trust what my options are. She has been supportive and empathic. I know she cares about my welfare, and yes, she is in HR. 'It's probably obvious, but I'm at the end of my tether . . . I think I need a fresh start away from all this,' I write.

My mental state is dire. The only reason I don't admit myself into Ward 17 is that Belle is recovering from major surgery in Hobart to realign her jaw, her final cleft palate operation.

I draft bullet points for Mary on why I need to leave Reuters:

- *The last time I had major mental health issues unrelated to Reuters was the 10th anniversary of the deaths of Namir and Saeed nearly 2½ years ago. My Reuters trauma is 'stuck', 'locked' in my body.*
- *Dee says I'm in an abusive relationship with an organisation that is omnipresent in my life.*
- *Not being told about the Toronto meeting shows Reuters isn't serious about putting in place lasting mental health strategies and institutionalising my role.*
- *What I saw in the president's office proved the company's culture won't change.*
- *I want to work with people I like and respect, who genuinely care about mental health.*

Days, maybe a week later, I speak to my HR friend again, who has spoken to members of the leadership. If I stay my work will be run through a journalists' council I'd be part of, effectively stopping me contacting the leadership directly.

Mary listens quietly as I list the reasons I need to quit. She sits on the couch in the living room, staring out the window as I read from my note. Mary says she understands but then awkward silence separates us. Privately, she is bewildered at how fast things spiralled downward following my overseas trip and afraid for our family's financial stability. She gets up and leaves the room.

PART FOUR

PART FOUR

19

Writing a new narrative

I grieve and mourn a career that has spanned half my life. I'm humbled by kind messages from colleagues when my departure is announced in January 2020. I've learnt that you need to take charge of your mental health, I write in a farewell message. Educate yourself. Find out what works. Getting help is strength, not weakness.

Mary and I also are dealing with some family challenges: Belle was diagnosed with PTSD last month, a result of the abuse and neglect she suffered in the Jakarta orphanage. It's a relief in some ways. Many things fall into place. The diagnosis makes sense to Belle, who now has context for her journey. She hires a personal trainer, gets contact lenses, has her hair dyed blue, buys new clothes, and plans her next tattoo. The ink on Belle's arms, shoulders and back reflect her Indonesian heritage, her love of animals and birds, as well as her mental health. I never imagined Belle and I would share the same tattoo artist, a former bikie named Avery who has a long ginger beard.

Belle has turned to me in recent weeks with a smile: 'I know I've said this already today, but I'm happy.' My heart sings.

Patrick then survives a cardiac arrest at home in February and the overwhelmed emergency department at Launceston General Hospital can't work out what's wrong. Staff want to send him home. I confront doctors and interns in the middle of the ED on day two of Patrick's admission, telling them the situation is unacceptable: 'Google my name and see where I've been!' I say with controlled fury. I want them to understand I won't stop fighting for my son. Propped up in a nearby bed and attached to a machine monitoring his heart, Patrick is embarrassed by the fuss. The ED is full of sick people and no one else is giving the doctors a spray.

'Is Bogan famous?' Patrick asks Mary, using his nickname for me. He thinks I'm rough around the edges because of the casual way I dress, shouting at the TV when the rugby league is on. He paints, listens to classical music and podcasts about ancient history.

'No, but he knows how to throw his weight around,' Mary replies.

Days later, cardiologists at the Hobart Private Hospital diagnose Patrick with Long QT syndrome, a disorder of the heart's electrical activity that is usually inherited. It's a relatively common cause of sudden death in children and young adults. The cardiologists fit Patrick with an implantable cardioverter-defibrillator (ICD).

It's a traumatic time for the whole family. Months later, Belle and Patrick are feeling better. I'm still largely off social media. Sometimes I sit and think about nothing, I look out the living room at the South Esk River and the Great Western Tiers. I don't listen to the radio or watch the news much. I might read something interesting, and my mind repays me with insight because my head isn't overcrowded. My wonderful HR colleague who arranged my exit from Reuters ensured I got a generous payout beyond the company's legal obligation, so I'm under no financial pressure. I've paused writing this memoir. I want to let things settle for a while.

I've started collaborating with Dr Sadhbh Joyce, a clinical neuropsychologist who has done ground-breaking research on workplace mental health at the Black Dog Institute. We plan to develop a blueprint for organisations we believe will reduce suffering in the workplace. I met Sadhbh (pronounced Sive) a few years earlier when Reuters agreed to use a company Sadhbh and her partner Jamie Watson run called Mindarma that offers online resilience training for employees. Sadhbh also treats people with work-related psychological injury in private practice in Sydney.

Sadhbh and I have different backgrounds that make for a great partnership. Born and raised in west Ireland, Sadhbh has an innate understanding of trauma. She has lived experience of burnout.

One day, after a lengthy chat with Steve Biddulph, I tell Mary I'm deliberately delaying the work I need to do on my emotions. Mary nods. She's known this for a long time. So have all my good clinicians. Steve has even tried to engage me on my feelings.

It was a simple rule where I grew up in the small New South Wales country town of Portland. Boys didn't cry. I fitted in well at primary school, played cricket in summer and rugby league in winter. Both sports frightened me a bit, but country boys had to be tough. Unfortunately, I was athletic and fast, so coaches put me near the action. But it was more than that. I was raised in a home where emotions weren't expressed. My mother had another son who died several hours after birth in a Sydney hospital when I was two. Mum had gone to Sydney because of complications during pregnancy. This was the biggest trauma in my parents' lives but Mum 'just got on with it', she told me 50 years later. After being sexually abused at nine by a relative and never telling anyone, coping was second nature to Mum. I don't recall much affection between my parents, or to my younger sister Holly and me when we were children. Dad, an electrician, would come home from work in his overalls and boots, grab a beer and spend time in his vegetable garden. He drank a lot, but never shouted or was violent. If he argued with Mum, he'd fly up the dirt lane in his ute to a local pub.

Generations of men have grown up unable to feel because they never saw any closeness between their parents, says Steve.

—

Determined to dig into the emotions of the past, I turn first to the Bali bombings. As I comb through Reuters articles I wrote from Kuta Beach eighteen years earlier, Hanabeth Luke's name jumps out. Hanabeth, 22, was in the Sari Club with her boyfriend, Marc Gajardo, when the car bomb exploded outside. Marc was killed. Did I interview this young Australian woman, this survivor of the attacks? It looks like I spoke to her near the ruins of the Sari the following day. What's wrong with my memory?

An iconic photo taken just after the bombings shows a barefooted Hanabeth in suede shorts and a black singlet top helping Australian Tom Singer, seventeen, escape. Flames engulf a minivan metres away. Tom, wearing only boardshorts, was severely burned and died a month later. Australian media called Hanabeth 'the

Angel of Bali'. Hanabeth became an anti-war activist. She urged British Prime Minister Tony Blair during a televised forum not to send troops to invade Iraq in 2003. Hanabeth published a memoir called *Shock Waves: Finding Peace After the Bali Bomb* to mark the tenth anniversary of the attacks. Since 2011, Dr Hanabeth Luke has been a lecturer at Southern Cross University's School of Environment, Science and Engineering.

Hanabeth has made her life count. But did I really meet her? Would she remember me? Her email address is on her university profile page.

'Hi Hanabeth – This might seem like a strange voice from the past . . .'

I send the email on a Friday. The following Monday I'm driving home after dropping Harry at school when my phone rings and goes to voicemail. I don't recognise the number. I play the message when I get home:

'Hi Dean, it's Hanabeth. Thanks for the email. I just thought I'd give you a buzz.'

My chest tightens. What the fuck is going on?

I make a cup of tea, get my notepad, take a few deep breaths. Hanabeth sounds relaxed. I'm not, though as usual I can keep the anxiety out of my voice. I ask Hanabeth about her life before getting to my crucial question: does she remember talking to me?

'Of course, you saw me and came over and asked if I was involved. I just told my story . . . After you I spoke to other journalists.'

She remembers things so clearly. Why had I forgotten?

'It must be hard for journalists, people unloading on you,' she says.

'We were never trained for dealing with the consequences of what we witnessed, talking to survivors,' I reply.

I sense Hanabeth has made peace with her past. Her voice is breezy. She has a husband, two children, aged five and three.

Police hadn't cordoned off the ruins of the Sari Club when I arrived less than twelve hours after the attacks, so I went over for a closer look, heart racing. A white L300 Mitsubishi minivan detonated outside as the club heaved with young backpackers and surfers from around the world. Ever since, no matter where I am, I say the words L300 under my breath in Indonesian when I see a white Mitsubishi minivan. I look for the boxy shape and the Japanese carmaker's three-diamond logo.

It didn't register I was treading on the edge of a crime scene that should have been swarming with investigators. I was the only one on it. Fire crews had extinguished the inferno, but wisps of smoke rose from the ashes. An acrid taste invaded my mouth, my nostrils. I was afraid of smelling flesh. My foot disturbed a piece of wood, revealing a bloodied hand, palm down, shorn off at the wrist. I kept moving.

Something then stopped me in my tracks. *Evil.* There was a formless presence from the ruins to the street. I could feel it, almost touch it. I'd read about survivors who say evil visits the site of a manmade atrocity. I wasn't religious or spiritual, I was a methodical news agency journalist who did one story and moved on to the next. I believed in what I could see. But there was evil there. It's a sensation I never experienced again.

I took a taxi to the main hospital in Denpasar, Bali's capital. I rushed to the doors but stopped to allow nurses pushing a foreigner on a gurney to enter. The young man was probably in his early twenties, but his entire face was burned, so it was hard to tell. A white sheet covered the rest of his body. He stared silently at the ceiling. I froze. I'd never seen a burns victim. My stomach clenched; I felt like a voyeur. *I shouldn't be here. I can't intrude given what these people are going through.* I moved away from the entrance, where I wouldn't be noticed. It was remarkably quiet because everyone was inside the 770-bed Sanglah hospital.

My job was simple – go into the public wards where rows of burned and maimed survivors lay, some alone, others comforted by family or friends, and get their story. Indonesian hospitals had little security, and I could talk my way past just about anyone.

But I couldn't do my job. I didn't even know what questions to ask. *What if family members get angry, call me a vulture? Is that what I am?*

Years later I think a part of me would have struggled to cope with the distress inside. I didn't have the emotional tools to deal with such grief. But the biggest obstacle at that moment was confusion, or was it shame? My identity was at stake. In that moment, I didn't want to be a journalist. Or I didn't know how.

I couldn't go to the hospital morgue either, which was full of bodies charred beyond recognition, wrapped in white sheets. Many more lay in a courtyard at the back of the hospital. Because I couldn't go through the front doors, I didn't see a large notice-board inside with pages of names stuck to it. A page for each letter in the alphabet, people reported missing by relatives and friends from all over the world – crucial details for any news story. I didn't speak to a single person.

My mind warred with itself for 15–20 minutes, then I took a taxi back to Kuta Beach.

That was the biggest story of my life at the time. It was nearly fifteen years before I told Mary what happened. Longer to understand why.

On my way to Kuta, another Reuters reporter, Joanne Collins, an Australian, arrived from Jakarta and called me asking what she should do. Go to the hospital, Jo, I said. Get quotes and details from survivors and family members. I'll stay at the bomb site because senior officials should arrive soon. I didn't tell Jo I had just been at the hospital. It had been less than a year since Jo experienced horrible loss. She and Reuters cameraman Harry Burton had planned to get married. Gunmen claiming to be Taliban murdered Harry in Afghanistan on 19 November 2001. Mary and I named our son Harry in honour of our Tasmanian friend.

That evening I lay on a big bed at the Hard Rock Hotel Bali, a short walk from the bomb site. It was 8 or 9 pm. I think the Reuters team was staying at the hotel, but I didn't get everyone together. I should have had the text journalists, photographers and camera operators planning coverage for the next day (I was deputy bureau chief for Indonesia). My mind wandered as I stared at the ceiling.

Years later I recall a weird sensation in my body as I lay on that bed. I think my body was trying to do something: shake, shiver, sweat. I'm not sure, but I suspect trauma was trying to escape. I was a failure for not entering the hospital. I grieved for the Balinese. My luxurious hotel room insulted the dead, the survivors and their families.

I now know what it was that cut me to the bone all those years ago – I dishonoured the survivors by not telling their story. By not doing my job. That was my shame. Sure, some people don't want to talk to journalists in such a situation. But many do. They want the world to know what happened and as a journalist you can give them the choice.

When I look back over my career, I can't recall anyone in crisis saying no to me. I interviewed a US veteran on camera inside the grounds of the War Remnants Museum in Ho Chi Minh City who couldn't stop crying. Graphic exhibits and photographs, including of the My Lai massacre, showed the horrors the Vietnamese suffered. It was 1998 or 1999, and this veteran's first trip back. He insisted we keep filming.

I'm also reminded of what Cait McMahon from the Dart Center said several years ago, how some journalists didn't know whether to act as a reporter or a person when covering traumatic events. Those who were confused about their role had the highest post-trauma reactions, Cait's research had shown.

'It seems it doesn't matter which way you go as long as you're clear and feel good about your decision. It's the ambivalence that can be your undoing,' Cait had said.

I've wondered if this made me more vulnerable. I spent nearly a week in Bali churning out story after story but still didn't go to the hospital. It was the only time I ever felt conflicted about my role to bear witness.

When I next see my psychologist Dee Cooper, I recognise the emotions in my body as we talk about Bali.

'You dissociated there,' she says. 'You checked out, split off what happened and ended up with memory fragments you never processed, never integrated into your life, until now.'

Tears well in my eyes. My whole body feels hot. I sit with the sensation. I'm okay with it.

I struggle a bit for a month as I go through the old Bali material. But writing down my thoughts helps. So does allowing the experience to roam my mind during my walks, while I'm driving or talking with Mary.

In a later session, Dee asks me to consider my mental state when I got to the Sanglah hospital. I think back: I'd reported the story from home in Jakarta that night, was in the newsroom for hours, went to the airport, no sleep, flew to Bali, then to the bomb site. Maybe it wasn't humanly possible to enter the wards, I say. And you didn't know how to sit with those people, adds Dee. The final piece to Bali is in place and it's not what I expect: I show myself compassion.

—

Steve Biddulph writes in his latest book *Fully Human* how emotions are as important to humans as breathing and walking, that they smooth out and resolve anxieties and fears so we can return to balance. That's what I can feel happening in my mind and body these past few months. Balance, a sense of equilibrium. Calmness. Emotions occur naturally. Tears fill my eyes as I write a social media post for Namir and Saeed to mark the thirteenth anniversary of their deaths on 12 July 2020. My joy listening to Harry and his band from school, Frogs in Suits, practise in the shed, then play their first gig at a pub in Launceston. I can hold Mary fully when she gets burnout at the end of the year and quits her job. I swell with pride as Patrick, his chest attached to cables, pounds a treadmill in his cardiologist's heart clinic, testing his defibrillator for the first time. For Belle when she says she wants to study full-time to get qualifications in hospitality.

I'm talking to Dee one day when she says psychologists often ask why trauma is so sticky for some people. There are those who get through with only minor impact while others have it in their DNA to manage, Dee says.

'Then there are people like you, Dean, who had this titanium around them,' Dee adds. 'That's when we look at early development, where there might be a stickiness around trauma. You grew up where there was no abuse but in a family where the emotional quotient wasn't nurtured.'

Dee says that when Namir and Saeed were killed, I went into a state of 'dead calm'. 'Your default mechanism was coping. Other people at various times in your place would have said, "Enough, I'm leaving." You coped.'

In Ward 17 during my first admission, Maryam asked me to write for her why I didn't cry. I usually typed plenty when she gave me homework; not this time. After recounting how my Lebanese colleague Mariam Karouny rescued me when I wept in Baghdad, I wrote:

'I've always been the rock for people, the cool head, the one who got things done without collapsing in a heap . . . So why can't I cry? Detachment? Numbness? Don't want to show weakness? Conditioned this way (Mum)?'

Maryam gave two reasons: 1) survival mechanism and 2) my mother. After reading my manuscript in 2022, Maryam added professional training. This had never occurred to me but cannot be underestimated. I'd call it professional training and support. From the moment I joined Reuters in 1993, the organisation made clear I had the potential to take on senior roles, bureau chief positions. I was given numerous opportunities, challenging assignments. I was mentored, did leadership training. Reuters equipped me with a lot of skills. And all my managers had my back, until I became damaged goods. My nature was to go the extra mile. And the company's commitment to me over more than two decades spurred me on.

All my good clinicians have zeroed in on my upbringing to explain why I went into emotional lockdown from Bali onwards, maybe even earlier in my career in Indonesia and Vietnam.

I've found it hard to accept this because I had it far better than most. My parents had little money but enough to give me a good education and get me to university. That's why I'm reluctant to attribute anything to them that might seem negative even if they gave me few emotional skills.

Dee says people like me also usually go to type with their life partners, seeking someone with that same titanium. I didn't with Mary, who combined toughness and independence with extraordinary softness and femininity.

——

Sadhbh and Jamie asked me earlier in the year if I wanted to host a mental health podcast for Mindarma. I jumped at the chance because I'd never done one. They wanted people in challenging occupations to talk about stress and trauma in their professional and personal lives. Super-organised Sadhbh gave me a list of people to interview.

First up is Tara Lal, a British-born firefighter from Sydney who published an extraordinary memoir in 2015 called *Standing on my Brother's Shoulders: Making Peace with Grief and Suicide.* Born in London, some of Tara's earliest memories were of the crippling mental illness her father had suffered all his life. When she was eight, Tara's mother was diagnosed with cancer and died five years later. At the time, Tara turned to her sensitive fifteen-year-old brother Adam for support. Adam was grieving silently, pouring his thoughts into his diaries. Four years after their mother died, in his first semester at Oxford University in 1988, Adam took his own life. Tara coped by keeping busy, by travelling, never stopping, until her family trauma caught up with her.

My challenge is to get Tara to explain in 30 minutes how her past has shaped who she is today: a firefighter, a researcher doing a PhD on how her workmates cope with the tragic suicides they encounter on the job, and a resilient woman with deep knowledge of trauma. I speak to Tara a few times to explain the aim of the podcast, get some background, and make her feel comfortable. I review other interviews she's done. I send her proposed questions so she can give me feedback. Then we set a date and record on Zoom. Sadhbh does an introduction, music is added. Sadhbh and I are delighted, Tara is natural and authentic. But what does Tara think?

'I am somewhat amazed to say that I love it,' she writes to us in an email. 'Amazed because I've never loved hearing myself speak, but I loved this. Your introduction Sadhbh, set the scene so perfectly and Dean, your questions enabled me to speak my "truth" in a way that I've never been invited to do before, and that brings me to tears (in a good way!).'

It doesn't get any better than that.

'Who am I now?' may be the most difficult and important question a veteran must finally answer, says psychotherapist Edward Tick in his book *War and the Soul*.

I suspect anyone who has suffered life-changing trauma confronts this dilemma. Six months after leaving Reuters, I can sense my new life narrative taking shape. I can feel the change emerging. I'm undergoing identity transformation, to use Tick's words. I can see five, even ten, years into the future, the books I'll write, the talks I'll give, the podcasts I'll present, the ferocious mental health advocate I'll become.

I do another seven podcasts for Mindarma over the coming months, including one with Guy 'Digger' Boland, an old mate from uni who barely survived a light plane crash in the northern

New South Wales town of Moree in 2011 that killed his parents, his older sister and the pilot. Digger's daughter Hannah was badly injured.

I was sitting at my desk in Singapore the day after the crash when my phone rang. It was Nick Todhunter, my closest friend from uni, calling from John Hunter Hospital in Newcastle where Digger was being treated. I hadn't seen Digger since Nick's wedding eighteen years earlier because I'd been overseas. But we'd been great friends. I put the phone down and got back to work. Digger would have 25 operations over the following years. I didn't call him, didn't visit. I was in a world of numbness.

Not long after my first Reuters special report was published in late 2016, Nick flew to Evandale. We went to Corinna, a small eco-retreat on the banks of the Pieman River in the Tarkine. Nick organised some friends including Digger to fly down a few months later. We stayed in the old miner's hut. There were only five bunks, so two of us took turns to sleep on the King Billy pine floor. Digger got a bunk each night because of the injuries he still carries, including blindness in one eye, partial sight in the other. He can't lift his arms above his shoulders. But with walking poles, Digger managed on the hikes since his upper body took most of the crash impact. In the hut, we played cards and laughed as we drank Tasmanian pinot noir and whisky. We feasted on beef ragu Nick cooked, as well as scotch fillet steaks fried on pans over the open fire.

I took my friends into the Tarkine again the following year. Tears were shed as we talked about our vulnerabilities and worries. A few of us braved the frigid waters of the Huskisson River for a swim, including Digger. He was the last to fly back to the mainland after that trip. As I drove him to the airport, I said: 'Mate, I let you down by not coming to see you after the crash. I am sorry. I was a shit friend.' Digger put his arm across my shoulder and said there was no need to apologise but that he understood.

Like I did with Tara, I spend time with Digger making sure he's prepared for the podcast. He's never really spoken publicly about the tragedy. During the interview, Digger talks about his darkest days and how he decided he was up for the fight of his life with support from his partner Fiona and his friends.

It's while preparing the podcast with Digger that I realise I'm still a journalist. I love talking to people like Tara and Digger and doing the research so they can share their stories. A big piece of my old identity is still there. I'm no longer damaged goods. What was once the foundation of my old self is part of my new narrative. My new identity.

20

Rules of engagement

My friend Peter Whish-Wilson, the Greens senator for Tasmania, drops by one weekend in early 2020. Peter and I met years ago and clicked the way some people do. We were both born in 1968, our kids are similar in age, and we share a passion for the Tarkine.

Peter and I often talk about the cost of war on civilians as well as veterans and their families. Peter served in the Australian army while I was at university. His father fought in Vietnam. Did two tours.

It's late summer as Peter and I catch up under the old walnut tree in my garden. Tasmania has largely escaped the bushfires ravaging eastern Australia, but we know it's just a reprieve after a record 210,000 hectares burned the previous summer. We chat for a bit, then Peter catches me off-guard by asking if I'd join the campaign to get Julian Assange out of London's Belmarsh prison and home to Australia.

Some people may find this hard to understand, but I haven't

paid much attention to Assange's fate in recent years, even after the Trump administration indicted him in 2019 for publishing the military and government secrets Chelsea Manning sent to WikiLeaks in 2010. Truthfully, there was little room in my head for the wider world when PTSD and moral injury overwhelmed me. And it's possible I subconsciously avoided thinking about Assange because he stood up for Namir and Saeed and I didn't.

I found a 10,000-word statement Manning read at her military trial in early 2013 while doing research for my book. It had been Manning's first opportunity to explain why she pulled off what was then the biggest leak of official secrets in US history.

Manning said the information would show the true cost of the Iraq and Afghanistan wars and hopefully spark debate about US military intervention abroad. She said analysis of the documents might make people re-evaluate counterterrorism and counter-insurgency operations that ignored the impact on affected communities. 'This is possibly one of the more significant documents of our time removing the fog of war and revealing the true nature of twenty-first century asymmetric warfare,' she wrote in a note to WikiLeaks accompanying the files.

Of the footage showing Namir and Saeed being killed, Manning told her court-martial hearing: 'I hoped that the public would be as alarmed as me about the conduct of the aerial weapons team crew members. I wanted the American public to know that not everyone in Iraq and Afghanistan are targets that needed to be neutralized.'

Manning was convicted of espionage and other offences and jailed for 35 years. President Barack Obama commuted Manning's sentence before he left office in early 2017, meaning she still served seven years, some in solitary confinement. Peter has been one of Assange's strongest supporters in Australia.

He tells me Trump's government has charged Assange under a World War One era law that has never been used against a journalist. It could set a precedent for Washington to indict reporters of any nationality, no matter where they live, for publishing classified information. Assange faces up to 175 years in prison. Peter is trying to get Australian journalists to speak up.

'How would you feel talking about Collateral Murder, why it was so important this footage be seen around the world? You could talk about the impact it's had on you, too,' Peter says.

'I know the video is distressing for you,' he adds gently. 'Don't feel pressured. If you can't do it, that's okay.'

Collateral Murder connects me to Assange and Manning by an invisible thread. Namir and Saeed would have been forgotten statistics of the Iraq War if not for them. The tape will keep the names of my colleagues alive forever.

I think for a few moments, then say: 'Peter, I'm fine talking about the footage. I'm just an old journo with PTSD living down here in Tasmania. Can I really help?'

'People need to be reminded of how significant that tape was,' Peter replies. 'Australians have forgotten what Julian's case is about. I think you can make a difference.'

I'll do it, I tell Peter.

Peter puts a seasoned *Guardian* journalist and columnist in Sydney called Paul Daley in touch with me. I'm sceptical Paul will find a story, but he says let's chat and we have a few conversations. Paul focuses on the briefing the two American generals gave me in Baghdad, gets me to walk him through the hour I spent in Saddam's former Republican Palace, watching the opening minutes of Collateral Murder. I've never gone into such detail before, even with Mary or Dr Maryam. Because I made peace with myself over Namir and Saeed nearly three years ago, I haven't thought much about the briefing since then. But Paul's probing lights a fire under me. The lying and deception by the US military come flooding back. I can now see the staggering hypocrisy of the American government charging Assange for showing the world what the war in Iraq really looked like.

I read the eighteen-count indictment for the first time, skimming through its 37 pages, searching for a reference to the tape. Huh. Not there. I get my highlighter and read the document more closely, several times. The indictment is an attempt to criminalise what journalists do getting information from sources and then publishing the material. The footage is not among the charges but the rules of engagement from 2006 to 2007 that WikiLeaks released on the same day as the video are. How can that be? Why isn't this tape that catapulted Assange into the international spotlight, made WikiLeaks a household name, the centrepiece of the indictment?

Collateral Murder was one of the greatest scoops in journalism of the past two decades. It and the ROEs are inextricably linked. After saving a copy of the tape, Manning told her court-martial that she searched for and found the ROEs, a 2007 flow chart outlining the chain of command for the use of force in Iraq and a laminated 'ROE Card' soldiers carried with them that summarised the rules.

Then I get it. The US government doesn't want the video in a courtroom. Too embarrassing. Potential war crimes and cruel pilot banter.

The Guardian publishes two stories by Paul on 15 June 2020. The stories are shared more than 10,000 times on social media from the *Guardian*'s website.

I was blunt with Paul about how Reuters failed Namir and

Saeed by not confronting the US military when the footage was released. Paul had this in his draft story, but *Guardian* lawyers were worried and wanted Paul to get comment from Reuters. All the bosses from that era had left, I told Paul. The current leadership won't know anything. To save time, Paul cut that from the text. On the same day his stories are published, I write in a Facebook post:

'It's time I spoke frankly about this. The reaction of Reuters to the release of the tape by Julian Assange was unacceptable. We should have publicly called out the US military for lying in the first place – for claiming in a statement on 13 July 2007, that Namir Noor-Eldeen and Saeed Chmagh were killed "during a firefight". We should have called out the US military's lack of transparency – for not handing over the tape despite our repeated requests for it. The leadership of Reuters at the time – I include myself in this – owed it to Namir and Saeed to hold the US military to account. We failed them.'

Assange's legal team contact me a few days later, asking if I'll give a written statement for his defence and be a witness at his extradition hearing in September. I agree.

I do media interviews and appear on panels where clips from Collateral Murder are played. I watch Namir and Saeed die again and again. For perhaps the first time, I let the emotion in my voice go. Inevitably, Paul's stories put the pilots of Crazy Horse 1–8 in the spotlight. While it doesn't happen on air, I get asked if they should be prosecuted. In my mind, the more important question is how to prosecute the architects of the invasion – George W. Bush, Dick Cheney, Donald Rumsfeld and co. The men responsible for an illegal and reckless invasion based on the lies that Saddam Hussein possessed weapons of mass destruction and had direct ties to al-Qaeda. The real criminals are the men who put the pilots of Crazy Horse 1–8 above the al-Amin neighbourhood in eastern Baghdad in the first place.

—

I've spent years thinking about this and it's hard to accept, but I understand why Crazy Horse 1–8 regarded the men that included Namir and Saeed as a threat to the 2nd Battalion, 16th Infantry Regiment when they spotted them. Violence had peaked in Iraq for the entire war only a few weeks earlier. Baghdad was the epicentre of this carnage. I don't like it, but I understand why the crew sought permission to open fire. I can see how the group fell under the definition of hostile intent as the threat of the imminent use of force. The men might have looked relaxed, but some were carrying weapons; the cameras carried by Namir and Saeed had genuinely been mistaken for guns; firefights across al-Amin that morning all made for a reasonable conclusion they would attack. Having covered the war from Baghdad at the time, it would be intellectually dishonest for me to argue otherwise.

But nothing excuses shooting Saeed and the minivan. That rule of engagement was explicit: 'Do not target or strike anyone who has surrendered or is out of combat due to sickness or wounds.' It was written on the ROE card given to US soldiers. Similarly, the Law of Armed Conflict does not allow combatants to shoot people who are surrendering or no longer pose a threat. The Geneva Conventions prohibit attacks on the wounded. Instead, Crazy Horse 1–8 fired 120 cannon shells at Saeed, the two bystanders who came to help him, and the Good Samaritan van driver.

When Assange released Collateral Murder in April 2010, the military said 'all evidence available' supported the conclusion that Crazy Horse 1–8 shot armed insurgents, even though Saeed had nothing in his hands and the van driver was unarmed. The other two men didn't appear to be carrying weapons, either. Then US Defense Secretary Robert Gates called the investigation 'very thorough'. He said soldiers were operating in 'split-second situations' and that 'these people [WikiLeaks] can put out anything they want, and they're never held accountable for it'.

The truth is that Saeed, badly wounded, tried to get up for three minutes in view of Crazy Horse 1–8. The crew literally begged him to pick up a weapon before eventually opening fire. Despite the obvious breach of the ROEs and international conventions, an AR 15–6 military investigation cleared the pilots. Among its findings: 'The AWT [air weapons team] accurately assessed that the criteria to find and terminate the threat to friendly forces were met in accordance with the law of armed conflict and rules of engagement.' The investigation was ratified on 21 July 2007, by the same brigadier-general who showed me the opening minutes of the footage four days later.

A day after Assange published Collateral Murder, a military spokesman for Central Command, which oversaw Middle East operations, said, 'There was never any attempt to cover up any aspect of this engagement.' In fact, the military's lying began when the lieutenant-colonel in Baghdad issued the statement that said Namir and Saeed were killed during a firefight. Officers in the 2–16 reviewed the video and audio recordings from Crazy Horse 1–8 several times after the attack. The military had time to work out its response. The lying continued when the brigadier-general outlined to me the military's so-called investigation. He said some of the men could 'clearly' be seen carrying RPGs before the Crazy Horse 1–8 crew had used the word RPG. And when he briefly mentioned the attack on the minivan, he said the driver was believed to be aiding insurgents, giving me a very limited account of that event. The Pentagon was deceitful in withholding the tape while I arranged for foreign media bureau chiefs in Baghdad to meet senior military officers to talk about journalist safety. It engaged in a cover-up by stonewalling Reuters' efforts to get the video for nearly three years.

When reporters in Washington asked a separate spokesman for Central Command where the tape was, he said the military couldn't find it. Another lie. Manning found it easily enough two months earlier. So did an officer in the 2–16 who showed it to a Reuters photographer called Carlos Barria in Baghdad in September 2007. Carlos, an Argentinian, had finished one embed with the military and been moved to the 2–16. Carlos went to the command post to introduce himself. A senior officer expressed surprise he was from Reuters. Didn't Carlos know the 2–16 was on the ground that day? Carlos had no idea. The military decided where to embed journalists, though it probably never occurred to anyone that putting Carlos in the 2–16 might be insensitive. The officer explained the context, then asked Carlos if he wanted to see the video. Confused, Carlos said sure. The officer opened his laptop and played the first few minutes, up to where Crazy Horse 1–8 opened fire. Carlos then called me.

Inevitably, the lying escalated to a US secretary of defence.

That's why the US government didn't put the tape in Assange's indictment – that snapshot of the war would have exposed the hypocrisy of its case against him.

Robert Gates claimed that watching the video was like looking at the war through 'a soda straw', there was no 'context or perspective'. I was the one who got the soda straw view – being shown less than three minutes of the tape without advance warning. I've often wondered if I was set up, the briefing choreographed. Why show any video to me at all? That was unusual. Was it planned so I'd go away with that image of Namir burned into my head, drop my investigation into why my staff were killed? And why did American troops turn up at Namir's family home in Mosul asking about non-existent ties to terrorists? Seeking dirt on Namir or his family? It was a febrile time in Washington. Iraq commander General David Petraeus was preparing to report to congress on his counterinsurgency strategy. It would be the most eagerly awaited testimony by a military leader in US history. The unlawful killing of journalists working for the foreign media in Baghdad might have tarnished the star performance he was to give.

That was one reason Collateral Murder was so powerful. It was pure truth-telling. No military officials could deflect, sanitise, provide 'context'. There is also no tape like it from any war in history in the public domain. The only comparable footage – the execution of a Vietcong prisoner on the streets of Saigon by South Vietnam's national police chief on 1 February 1968 – is held under licence by NBC and can be obtained only with special permission. Everyone remembers the Pulitzer Prize–winning photo by Eddie Adams. But not the footage because it's not a mouse-click away.

Adams's photo, taken at the start of the Tet Offensive, changed how Americans saw the war in Vietnam. It's part of the historical record. I doubt few people would argue his photo should never have been published. Or that the Associated Press should have censored it or given the US military, or its South Vietnamese allies, a chance to provide 'context'. A photo that shows Nguyen Van Lem's temple bulging as the bullet enters his head. The world needed to see the moment of Lem's death. The casual way he was executed.

Can the same be said for Collateral Murder? Absolutely. Americans had a right to know how their government was conducting war in Iraq. How their taxpayer money was being spent. The cost being imposed on Iraqis. So did the people of Australia, whose conservative government had eagerly followed Bush into Iraq. It was in the global public interest because up to that moment, so much of the war in Iraq was hidden from view. Collateral Murder runs a mere 38 minutes. But from the pilot chatter and the casual way permission was given to open fire, we can reasonably assume this was the everyday in Iraq and Afghanistan. The attack on the van was not out of the ordinary.

—

In September 2020, Assange's legal team twice tell me to get ready to give evidence by video link at his extradition hearing. Prosecutors acting for the US government might want to question me about my written statement for the defence.

I wear a tie and sit in front of my computer, adrenaline running through my body into the night. In the end, the prosecution doesn't contest my statement. Why? I don't know. But I don't get a chance to speak.

In January 2021, judge Vanessa Baraitser of the Westminster Magistrates' Court rules Assange a suicide risk if extradited to the United States but agrees with every point in the prosecution's case. In Washington, Donald Trump reluctantly leaves the White House. Joe Biden is the new American president. But Biden won't drop the charges. His government appeals. Collateral Murder and the leaked classified documents, I suspect, embodied an act of whistleblowing and publishing that threatened US power to its very core, no matter who is in office. An example must be made of Assange.

It also dawns on me that if I'd watched Collateral Murder years earlier, I probably would have gotten the sequence right and stopped blaming Namir. I'd have seen Crazy Horse 1–8 get permission to open fire before Namir peered round that corner. Maybe I wouldn't have been such a coward. I might have demanded a strong public response from Reuters, an independent investigation. Instead, I stood by as Reuters let the United States off the hook. Because I liked and respected my Iraqi colleagues so much, that made it harder to have failed them. I wasn't the bureau chief I thought I was in their eyes. That was part of my moral injury.

The strange thing is, and maybe it's not strange, I don't lose sleep over this revelation. It's just part of my narrative now, my story.

21

Fear, not what I expected

When people ask how I'm doing, I usually say 'I'm really good' or 'Mentally, I'm the best I've been in years'. I get a bit of anxiety but no flashbacks. I have only the occasional nightmare. My concentration levels are back to full-strength. In May 2021, I told my psychologist Dee Cooper I felt good. Dee said I have a 'big picture level of peace' but things will still break off and affect me.

A few weeks later I had a rare nightmare about the Bali bombings. Why? No idea except I'd been stressed that day about various things. Psychologist Wendy Gall was the first clinician to advise me to be a journalist when I woke after a nightmare. Finish the story, give it an ending, she said. With Bali that morning, I went through the therapy I'd done and noted the bombings happened nearly two decades ago. I concluded the story.

My biggest problem is unexpected noise. I still jump out of my skin if Lois barks suddenly or a door is slammed. This classic PTSD arousal symptom is impervious to my years of therapy.

I've never really delved into the reasons behind my noise sensitivity. I just put it down to all the explosions I heard and felt in Baghdad, car bombs rattling the office windows, that sort of thing. It's only when I read *The Evil Hours: A Biography of Post-Traumatic Stress Disorder* by David J Morris for a third time in October 2021, that it falls into place. A former US Marine turned journalist, Morris reported on the Iraq War until an IED exploded under his US Humvee in Baghdad in 2007. It was a lucky escape for Morris and the soldiers inside. 'During my worst times post-Iraq, times when I felt the most alienated and angry at the world, it felt like my body was back in Dora [a Baghdad suburb] and Ramadi, places where I lived on a knife-edge of fear for weeks at a time,' Morris writes. 'It was, in short, a cumulative feeling of stress and fear that came back to me, not unresolved memories relating to a specific close call.'

That's it! I lived on a knife-edge *every day* in Baghdad. It doesn't cross my mind that my knife-edge has been my family's eggshells. I tell Mary I think I finally understand why I'm still so jumpy. I was never kidnapped, but it could have happened. It was always at the back of my mind. Never blown up, but riding in the old, armoured BMW with an Irish bodyguard . . . Same for insurgents raiding the office or a mortar landing. The Iranian-made rocket that hit the roof of the BBC house across the narrow road from us in May 2008 hurt no one, thankfully, but scared us half to death. More staff could have been killed while covering stories. In my performance review for that year, I used typical news agency brevity to describe the risk: 'While a number of Iraqi staff were lightly wounded in various incidents in 2008, no one was hurt seriously. No one was killed.'

My body inhabited a state of constant fear during the roughly 700 days and nights I spent in Iraq. All that energy got stored and has never been released. I reckon this explains why my most frequent nightmare was being chased by gunmen through the streets of Baghdad, getting abducted. My autonomic nervous system (ANS) has been aroused since I left Baghdad, and new stresses – unexpected noise – push it higher. The fear in my body from Iraq gets confused with everything around me, like Lois barking. Patrick and Belle, now 21, and Harry, 19, don't notice as much. But Mary does; she rides the rollercoaster of every incident.

'In PTSD the body continues to defend against a threat that belongs to the past. Healing from PTSD means being able to terminate this continued stress mobilization and restore the entire organism to safety,' says Bessel van der Kolk in *The Body Keeps the Score*. In late 2021 I decide it's time to get to grips with the Polyvagal Theory, something that excites van der Kolk.

Stephen Porges, a neuroscientist and professor of psychiatry at the University of North Carolina, introduced the Polyvagal Theory in 1994. Polyvagal refers to the branches of the vagus nerve that travels through much of the body, connecting vital organs such as the brain, lungs, heart and stomach. The Polyvagal Theory provided a more sophisticated understanding of the ANS. Or, as van der Kolk writes, 'the biology of safety and danger, one based on the subtle interplay between the visceral experiences of our own bodies and the voices and faces of the people around us. It explained why a kind face or a soothing tone of voice can dramatically alter the way we feel. It clarified why knowing that we are seen and heard by the important people in our lives can make us feel calm and safe, and why being ignored or dismissed can precipitate rage reactions or mental collapse.' (Managers, did you read that?)

I've instinctively wanted Mary to soothe me more. Mary in turn has wanted to feel safer around me. Neither can happen with a 53-year-old man on edge in the house. Whenever we feel threatened, we call for help, support and comfort, van der Kolk says. If that doesn't happen, we revert to fight, flight or freeze. I rage: Mary shuts down. I don't get soothed: Mary feels unsafe. The cycle never stops because fear is locked in my body.

I share these new thoughts and ideas with Mary. She nods. It's a momentous moment. I want to be able to soothe you, Mary says in the following days. You need to feel safe first, I reply. Maybe we *can* figure this out.

—

Dee is delighted when I tell her I get the Polyvagal Theory. And she agrees that fear from Baghdad is trapped in my body. The validation is immense.

'The definition of PTSD can be very limiting for some people,' Dee adds.

'How do I deal with this?' I ask.

'We go back to EMDR,' she says.

'Does that work for something that *didn't* happen?'

'I believe it will,' Dee replies. She tells me that next session we'll focus on a moment when I felt really terrified in Iraq.

On cue, the US soldier pointing his M249 squad automatic weapon at me pops into my head, adrenaline surges through my body. What seems like yesterday was eighteen years ago.

Two weeks later, I sit opposite Dee. She asks me to take several deep breaths and to update her on how my body reacts. She will stop if I appear distressed. And she wants me to have a safe space in my head if I need somewhere to go. I choose the Tarkine rainforest.

My chest tightening, I recount an experience that lasted a few minutes: We've come to the exit of the military base in Baghdad, not the entrance. I order my Iraqi driver to stop. There is a soldier behind sandbags, hunched over a machine gun aimed at our windscreen. Don't move, I tell the driver.

My body is heating up, head to toes.

'Go slowly,' says Dee. 'Breathe. Find the image that is the worst moment in this memory.'

I open the car door, hold up my blue PRESS flak jacket, and get out. I yell 'media' and 'journalist', but the soldier says nothing. I walk towards him slowly, left hand raised, the other holding the flak jacket so he can see the PRESS sign in fluorescent white.

'Hey, mate! I'm a journalist!'

He's twenty metres away.

'Fuck man, I nearly lit you up!' he shouts.

I'm sweating now, getting a headache, I tell Dee.

Dee moves her chair close to me. 'When you look at this worst moment, what is the emotion that goes with the image?' she asks.

I pause. 'It wasn't emotion, more a crystal-clear understanding that I had to do something. Take responsibility. If we reversed, the soldier might shoot, think we're suicide bombers who've changed their minds'

'So that means you could have died.'

Dee asks me to rate my distress when I think about this on a scale of 0–10.

Ten.

Okay, Dee says, hold that thought: 'Your belief in this moment is that *I have to take responsibility.* Is there a connection to not feeling safe in this situation? As you look at that image, noticing the thought that "I am responsible, I could die", be aware of that feeling in your chest, the heat in your body – and now follow my fingers.'

Dee puts her index and middle finger together in front of my face and moves them side to side, quicker than I expected, for about 30 seconds. It's slightly hard to follow the movement and hold the thought.

We do this a few times, with Dee asking how my body feels, to check how it is processing the felt impact of the trauma.

'How would you categorise the experience?' asks Dee.

'It was a close call. This sort of thing happened often to journalists in Iraq,' I say.

'It was a close call, but you made it,' says Dee.

Hold that thought, she tells me, then she moves her fingers in front of my face, a bit slower this time.

My body is cooling, I tell Dee. Tension is leaving my shoulders. Dee asks about my level of distress out of ten. It's dropping fast.

'Good,' she says. 'Now, what's important to take away from this? What do you believe about yourself as you reflect on that memory?'

I'm not sure, so Dee helps me.

'You're safe now,' she says gently.

Of course!

Hold that thought, Dee says again, moving her fingers slowly across my face.

'What can you see of that moment in Baghdad now?' she asks.

The scene is fuzzy. What had been a high-resolution photograph is blurry, vague, like the picture has gotten lost somewhere in my mind.

'You know Dee, I think this memory has just been folded and put in my linen cupboard,' I say, amazed.

'Try to recall it,' says Dee.

All I get is grey outlines.

By the time I get home, my headache is gone.

Mary is stunned when I tell her what happened. For the next two weeks, I don't blow up over Lois. I walk her every morning rather than curse her existence. I go off sugar. I'm less jumpy, less reactive to unexpected noise.

Sitting with Dee in March 2022, she gets up to close her window one morning. The noise outside is bothering me, she says. I hadn't noticed, I reply. We look at each other, eyes widening.

22

What is trauma?

Dr Maryam wrote in her notes after our first session in 2016 that I'd accepted my PTSD diagnosis, but the fact I never had what I considered a near-death experience bothered me until I understood what fear from Iraq had done to me. I spent most of my time behind concrete blast walls in Baghdad. It's only since I've understood the fear component that I've truly been able to accept my diagnosis.

The *DSM-5* says trauma must involve real or threatened death, severe injury or sexual assault such as rape to be called PTSD. Like my psychologist Dee Cooper said, this can be limiting for some even though PTSD is the lingua franca of trauma.

In Aceh I saw thousands of dead bodies along 250 kilometres of coastline after the Boxing Day tsunami, but never needed a single session of therapy on the tragedy. People are surprised when I tell them this. The final toll of dead and missing was 166,000; across a dozen countries around the Indian Ocean, 226,000. Manmade atrocities and personal violence are harder to deal with than acts of Mother Nature, experts say. But this was one of the biggest natural disasters in history. I saw the faces of Patrick and Belle everywhere I went in Aceh. It made the story deeply personal. In one photo I treasure, smiling boys at a camp for displaced people crowd around me, laughing with this pale, skinny foreigner. Yes, Aceh affected me. I got flashbacks, but they faded years ago.

I've concluded that the trauma experience is highly subjective, influenced by how we perceive our actions – and those of others – in relation to the event. I was proud of the work I did in Aceh and the way Reuters threw everything at the story, not just in the initial weeks, but for at least a year. I returned to Aceh six months after the tsunami to report on reconstruction efforts and how people were doing, navigating boggy roads down the coast with a photographer. We did the same trip at the one-year anniversary mark.

I believe my reporting in Aceh minimised the trauma impact on me. I've worked hard all my life but in Aceh I did so with a passion and urgency I don't think I ever matched. People with a car or motorbike stopped if they saw me hitchhiking in Banda Aceh (there was little fuel, making it hard to hire vehicles). No one accepted money, one young man said the world needed to know what had happened. Aid workers thanked me for what the media was doing. I had clarity about my role, unlike outside the Sanglah Hospital in Bali: I knew my job in Aceh was to bear witness, report the hell out of the story.

Late on New Year's Eve 2004, I got a message to call Paul Holmes, then the Reuters political and general news editor in New York. It had been another harrowing day for our team of a dozen reporters, photographers and cameramen. When I reached Paul on my satellite phone, he said the company was proud of our work, tell everyone we're thinking of them. Paul had gotten a list of Reuters journalists covering the tsunami across Asia and tried to contact them all. This wasn't standard practice, journalists got on with the job. But Paul had seen war and suffering during decades in the field. His call meant more to me than any I got in my 26 years at Reuters.

Trauma has affected many journalists I know in ways that fall outside the standard definition of PTSD.

Caroline Hawley was a BBC correspondent in Baghdad from the US-led invasion in March 2003 to early 2006. On 9 November 2005, she was in Amman with my friend Luke Baker, a Reuters journalist who spent years working in the Middle East and Africa. The Jordanian capital then was the last stop to Baghdad on the way in and the first stop on the way out. Caroline and Luke had just sat down in a restaurant on the lower ground floor of the Hyatt Hotel when a suicide bomber blew himself up in the lobby, one floor above. It was one of three coordinated suicide attacks in luxury hotels in Amman that night that killed 60 people and wounded 115.

The sound was deafening, Caroline later wrote to a colleague. 'I snapped my head around to see a column of fire and smoke on the stairway.' Caroline and Luke escaped unhurt. But Caroline would be haunted by what she didn't do soon after, when she and Luke returned to the hotel to report on what had happened. 'I saw bloodied bodies. Or were they still just about alive? I'll never know,' she wrote to her colleague. Rather than helping the wounded, Caroline said she ran to find ambulances.

'It was a relief to get away from all the blood. But why didn't I think to put [the wounded] in the recovery position first? In the shock of it all, I seemed to have forgotten the elementary rules of first aid.'

Caroline's breaking point came a few months later, when she

went back to Amman in March 2006 to make a documentary about the bombings. As she walked into the Hyatt, she felt a strange sensation in her left leg. It was the first trigger of what was later diagnosed as PTSD. Despite all the violence she saw and the danger she faced in Iraq, it was not helping those wounded people that troubled Caroline most. That, and getting world-class treatment for her PTSD.

'I remember feeling even worse about myself in my first treatment session – what right did I have to be sitting in a swanky [London] office getting help when so many Iraqis needed it more and would never, ever get it,' Caroline told me in late 2016.

I remember thinking, gosh, that sounds like moral injury. Of course, I wasn't about to tell Caroline that her psych had gotten it wrong. It just underscores the subjective nature of trauma and perhaps the failure of PTSD to capture this.

Mary has never been diagnosed with PTSD but is still troubled by what she witnessed as a journalist. Her worst memory, the image that can jolt her awake in the early hours and leave her frozen under the doona, condemning herself over and over: watching a young student shot by Indonesian security forces lying on the ground in front of a line of demonstrators, probably bleeding out. It was 1998 in Jakarta and students had brought the young man to the protest site for everyone to see. He might have been shot nearby. Mary is not sure. He was alive, barely. Working as a TV producer for Reuters, Mary watched from a small distance away. For 25 years she has wrestled with not helping the student, not trying to stop him bleeding, though that would have meant removing her shirt in a Muslim country. Did the student live or die? Mary tried without success to find out in early 2022. That experience broke her heart.

—

What I like about moral injury as a term is that the individual has agency, a say in what ails them. With PTSD, you are more of a victim, a passive participant in your diagnosis. PTSD doesn't capture the moral dimension of trauma. It also fails entirely to recognise endemic organisational and system betrayal, the callous workers' compensation system, the abuse that follows the initial trauma. Moral injury does.

A review in early 2019 of more than 100 scientific studies (Brett Litz was an author) showed moral injury might be conceptualised as: (a) the extent to which individuals assessed themselves as having committed moral violations, leading to perpetration-based symptoms; and (b) assessed themselves as victims of another's transgressive behaviour, leading to betrayal-based problems. (The review showed moral injury had been applied to healthcare providers, educators, law enforcement, child protection services and refugees.)

Moral injury was first described in Australia in 2015 by clinicians Zachary Steel and Dominic Hilbrink in their work with first responders and veterans. Think of firefighters who can't get close enough to pull people from burning homes but believe they should have; paramedics who tell themselves they could have gotten to car accidents faster; the scenarios with police officers are endless.

During my second Ward 17 admission, I was invited to speak to first responders and 000 operators who belong to the Code 9 Foundation. Code 9 supports current and retired personnel in Victoria with PTSD and their families. It has several thousand members. I spoke about the memorial service I was planning for Namir and Saeed the following week and my understanding of moral injury. Virtually none of the twenty people there had heard of moral injury, but the concept struck a chord.

One copper later told me he now understood why getting late to a domestic violence case years ago had so affected him.

After I spoke, I asked if anyone wanted to share a story. Another copper said his toughest role had been a dispatcher, sending colleagues into potentially dangerous situations with limited information. 'The worst part was the silence, not knowing what was happening,' he said. 'Were my colleagues okay?' A 000 operator said she couldn't get background screaming from calls she took out of her head. Most people probably wouldn't think of these situations if asked to describe PTSD.

The first evidence that journalists suffered moral injury emerged in 2017 when researchers found many members of the media who covered the 2015 refugee crisis in Europe suffered from what they witnessed. Journalists were shocked at having to carry bodies, including those of children, off beaches because there was no one else to do it. They questioned if they were doing enough while reporting the crisis. Should they stop and help people? They questioned the value of their work. And they felt shame at the behaviour of others such as local authorities.

Steel and Hilbrink put forward an expanded definition of moral injury – bearing witness to horror, situations dominated by inhumanity and gross injustice. I suspect many journalists would relate to this, as would people working in child protection, justice, legal, mental health, social welfare, politics, the environment and with refugees. The definition encapsulates the past 230 years for our First Nations people. 'This exposure to horror and malevolence creates a first-hand knowledge that destroys and pollutes the individual even though the individual in no way contributed to the atrocity and had no power to prevent it,' they wrote in an essay for a 2015 book called *Moral Injury: Unseen Wounds in an Age of Barbarism*. 'A threat to one's psychological integrity via an event that shatters one's sense of self, community, relationships and world order can have a profound effect on someone's sense of themselves in the world.'

Brett Litz and Patricia Kerig, a professor of clinical psychology at the University of Utah, wrote in 2019 that the notion people can suffer lasting damage from their own moral transgressions and from the actions of others was as old as humanity itself. The struggle for redemption and efforts to repair those harms were also central to the human story. It was only recently that these concepts had been considered clinically relevant social, biological and psychological problems, they said in the introduction to a special edition on moral injury in the *Journal of Traumatic Stress*.

They wrote of the centrality of moral judgements and decision-making that result in different outcomes. Moral challenges can lead to moral frustration: for moral stress, the outcome might be moral distress; and for a potentially moral injurious event, it might be moral injury after evidence of lasting impact was obtained. It's a bit like PTSD. Experiencing a traumatic event doesn't necessarily mean someone will get the condition, initial symptoms can pass. They must meet *DSM-5* criteria for a diagnosis.

Moral injury went somewhat mainstream when COVID-19 swept the world in 2020 because it captured the dilemma for overwhelmed hospital staff: who got a bed, who got ventilated, telling stricken families a loved one would die alone. Moral injury encapsulated the fury at hospital administrators and authorities for failing to provide enough personal protective equipment; at safety guidelines that contravened individual ethics. Media in Australia and the UK published harrowing accounts from inside hospitals from anonymous staff. Doctors and nurses in the United States were fired for speaking out publicly. The term moral injury, both types, appeared in news reports across the world: Litz's version where staff violated their own moral values for not doing enough and witnessing unimaginable suffering and death; and betrayal in a high-stakes situation that psychiatrist Jonathan Shay conceptualised from his work with American soldiers who fought in Vietnam.

In their 2019 paper, Litz and Kerig noted that for moral injury to be viable and useful, it needed to be defined as a reliably measurable syndrome. Have diagnostic criteria, like PTSD. Some experts say moral injury shouldn't be classified as a mental illness, that a 'normal' response to moral conflicts shouldn't be pathologised, characterised as psychologically abnormal. That trivialises moral injury. People want to know what's wrong with them and how to get help. I don't buy the notion that people dislike labels. What they hate is discrimination and prejudice from the workplace, insurance companies, government agencies, society at large. The harm from moral injury is deeply psychological, ruins relationships and can lead to suicide. Soldiers are trained to deal with danger on the battlefield. They suicide because of the guilt and shame they brought home from Iraq, Afghanistan, East Timor and Vietnam, from failed peacekeeping missions. From being abandoned by a country that sent them to war. I suspect countless people suffering workplace betrayal would benefit from understanding moral injury.

Dee sees moral injury among her first responder clients. It follows the initial trauma as an 'insult' to the PTSD. The workers' compensation process is a prime example. Workmates are often prohibited from speaking to their colleague on workers' comp, Dee says, which isolates the injured person, makes them feel abandoned and powerless.

'Everyone can see and feel PTSD, but moral injury sits in the context of a bigger structure of relationships: were you validated and kept safe?' she says. 'With moral injury, the system failed you. Has taken away your control.'

I've asked dozens of my veteran and first responder friends from Ward 17 what has been hardest to deal with: their original workplace trauma or abandonment by their organisations and then workers' comp/DVA hell? *Every single one* has said betrayal by their bosses and the organisations that were supposed to help them recover.

It's late one afternoon in April 2021. I'm so tired I want to drop to the floor and sleep. I've been working hard on the book and gone four days without sugar. I go to the takeaway shop in Evandale with Belle and buy three melting moment biscuits, two Florentine cookies and two Coke Zeros. I know, I know, I say to Belle. The sugar surge jerks me back to life.

I tell Mary I've softened over my former manager, who came out publicly in early 2021 as a transgender woman. I'd vowed to never speak to her again after what I saw as her failure to support me in my mental health role at Reuters. I admire her courage. She's gone through a years-long personal struggle I was unaware of. She is a human being, not a bureaucrat.

'I am very proud of you,' Mary says, hugging me.

My former boss looked after me at critical points in my life. I spoke openly to her about my trauma and treatment. I felt comfortable easing into work after my second and third Ward 17 admissions. When it came to my welfare and that of my family, she was a champion.

It took longer than I thought, but writing has also softened me. Writing has helped me heal. But as Mary jumped in and said, how Reuters treated me in 2016 was not okay. Then something extraordinary happens. The next day I feel that burden lift.

Mary had asked the night before if I was bitter about anything. Only 2016, I replied. Today, I'm not even sure about that. This is progress. Where is it coming from? Can you forgive an organisation? It's not like I've reached a point where it's time to get on with life. Reuters never accepted any responsibility, never apologised. I made clear to my kind HR colleague that I'd never sign anything if the company tried to muzzle me. And I still got a generous settlement. I was determined to control my truth.

Journal entry. Evandale, Tasmania, Apr 11, 2021: The burden has lifted. I've healed because I'm sharing my story. Communalising my trauma. This is significant. I feel lighter. For me it's not about forgiveness or saying it's time to get on with life fully. I'm so less consumed thinking about it. That means it's been integrated. Everyone is different, everyone's journey is different. How I was treated in the workplace mattered so much to me. I suspect it matters to many people. Leaving Reuters was key to my getting on with life. I was fortunate in being able to do that.

Later I'm listening to music by Tasmanian singer-songwriter Fiora as I walk around Evandale. Her music is a blend of dance, pop and electronic. Not my usual Foo Fighters, Smashing Pumpkins or Frogs in Suits. As I stride along breathing cool afternoon autumn air, noticing the patchwork of yellow and red leaves, Fiora drops the pace with a song that captures my state of mind: 'Let It Go By'. It's a sign, and possibly a new tattoo.

23

Recovery and reconnection

One of the challenges of trauma – mental illness in general, I suspect – is the word recovery. What does it mean? Recovery implies cured, fixed, good as new. Break your arm, it resets, you get normal use of the limb back. It's not like that with trauma, where you lose your identity, all sense of who you are. You freeze in time, but the years pass by.

I avoid using the word recovery because I don't think trauma has an end point. It's also not about returning to 'normal'. Traumatised people will never be the same. And that's okay because trauma makes living a fuller life possible. Viktor Frankl's book opened my mind to the prospect of finding meaning by raising awareness of PTSD. My heart and mind burst with enthusiasm. It was my first taste of post-traumatic growth.

Two clinicians and researchers from the University of North Carolina in Charlotte pioneered this concept in the mid-1990s. Richard G. Tedeschi and Lawrence Calhoun had observed changes in people after traumatic experiences that included new possibilities for life, better relationships, and a greater sense of personal strength and spiritual development. Tedeschi said he and Calhoun sought to focus on the aftermath of trauma rather than the event itself. I suspect post-traumatic growth is more likely when survivors have a strong support network.

One of my initiatives in the mental health role at Reuters was the use of storytelling to normalise the conversation around the topic. I wrote a few internal blogs, and then senior correspondents I knew wrote about their bipolar disorder (Mike Georgy in Beirut); being a mother running a big financial bureau and battling depression (Emma Thomasson in Berlin, on her previous posting to Zurich); newsroom burnout (Andy Cawthorne in Caracas); and the grief of losing a brother to cancer (Nidal al-Mughrabi in Gaza). In all, about 30 blogs circulated. They were a sledgehammer against stigma and shame in Reuters. They communalised what many individuals had suffered in silence. And they didn't cost the company a cent.

Andy told me he was 'astounded, a bit embarrassed, moved, concerned, happy at the torrent of feedback' he got from colleagues: half a dozen phone calls, 30 emails and about 20 direct messages on the company's editing system. 'Thanks for such an honest open blog. So many people across the company are struggling in the same way and it takes people like you, and Emma, to bring these issues into the open,' said one message.

The last blog I edited was by a TV producer in London called Ciara Lee. I didn't know Ciara, whose husband Eddy was queued behind stationary traffic on his motorbike in London when a van smashed into him in 2018. The driver wasn't paying attention. It took nine days for Eddy to die. All coma medication had to leave his system before he could be pronounced 'brain dead' and his body sent for organ donation. Eddy was 46. Ciara was 34.

They had a two-year-old son, Seren. Ciara emailed to say a
co-worker had given her one of my articles. After reading it,
Ciara wrote her own blog on the train to work.

I delayed opening Ciara's blog for days, knowing it would be
wrenching. When I did read her piece, what struck me was how
Ciara understood the connection between pain and hope and grief
and joy. She had captured the essence of *living* with trauma. And
she wasn't afraid to express it. Gosh, she will help people, I thought.

'The hardest moments in the following weeks and months
were those when I realised my brain might survive,' Ciara wrote.
'It wasn't going to break. I wasn't going to get respite from the
trauma around me. I had fantasised about being carried off to a
psychiatric hospital, strapped to a bed and drugged. I was being
forced to face the trauma, without anaesthetic . . .

'I will always be traumatised. It's part of who I am. But the most
important thing is I don't feel weakened by it. I am not fragile. My
mind feels stronger than ever. Every time I thought it was breaking, it was having its own workout. It was getting stronger.

'I still cry. I cry A LOT. I will always cry. I will always wish
I had died instead of Eddy that day. But I have clarity now.
A traumatised brain, in my opinion, can see things far more
clearly.

'I am sad, but I am also happy. I was so in love, but I am also
able to love again.'

Ciara contacted me in mid-2021 ahead of the third anniversary of Eddy's death. She wanted to write to him, but there was
nothing left to say other than note everything he'd missed. Ciara
had been reading about post-traumatic growth and thought she
was experiencing it. She had searched for normality but realised
her brain was now wired differently. She was happier achieving
something beyond normal.

'I feel far more deeply,' she wrote to me. 'I am sure it's why young widows and widowers often find love again, much to the horror of those around us. It's because we have an ability to feel the more intense emotions and not be afraid to act on them. Other than Seren's wellbeing, I feel almost no fear anymore.'

I know what Ciara means about fear. I have none except for my family's health. What can someone do to me that I haven't done to myself?

At home, I sense post-traumatic growth in greater calmness and balance in my life.

I've found more ways to enjoy time with my children, guide them on their own journeys. Belle once asked how I could possibly learn anything about PTSD from her. Easy, I said, rattling off three examples: she lives in the present; releases trauma through her body; and didn't take years to accept she had PTSD. It made her day, and mine.

Belle is a barista at cafes in Evandale and Launceston. Harry has taken a break from studying contemporary music at the University of Tasmania in Hobart to try to hit the big time with his band. I'm the manager. Patrick does some of the band's artwork. He is doing his Fine Arts degree while taking the odd commission for oil portraits.

My love, respect and admiration for Mary has reached new heights. We laugh and joke like we did in the old days. Watching TV shows and movies most nights unless Mary is doing a late shift as a support worker at a homeless shelter. Swapping books. Drinking rum and cokes at the Prince of Wales pub. Apologising to our friendly neighbours when our two goats Sassafras and

Wattle eat their flowers. We have also adopted two rescue grey-hounds, Harry and Rosie. Mary and I have grown together. We meet life's challenges as parents and a couple. There is genuine respect for each other and a shared commitment to provide a stable home for our children. Honesty has been vital as well as a willingness to keep having difficult conversations.

Mary has shown enormous patience. I've listened whenever she wants to vent about how hard it's been, although if I'm honest, a couple of times I wanted to say, 'Okay, I was a beyond-belief prick, but I don't want to talk about this anymore.' We enjoy each other's company. Talking about good times has helped us navigate tough ones because it reminds us why we got together in the first place. The richness of our experiences could never be replicated with someone else. What we have is worth fighting for.

Psychologist Dee Cooper reckons I'd become addicted to visiting sex workers. Dee's appraisal didn't surprise Mary, who got the PTSD part. She struggled with the emotionless, reckless and selfish side. I wasn't so sure about Dee's assessment. Visiting sex workers wasn't a compulsive habit, something I felt guilty or ashamed about immediately after, as per the definition of such addiction. It was often planned or opportunistic, entitled narcissistic behaviour.

I told Mary in 2022 I'd broken my promise to her in Starbucks in Singapore. I said I'd been faithful ever since I realised how deeply wrong my actions were, how much I'd hurt her.

Mary forgave me. She says she trusts me. And literally nothing has been left hanging in the air. At one point Mary made the comment that men and women weren't meant to be monoga-mous. Where is Mary going with this, I thought. So, I asked. Mary wanted to regain the intimacy I'd destroyed (my words) but didn't want to deprive (her words) me of sex in the mean-time. 'Did I still want to see sex workers?' she asked. I felt a physical stirring for a few seconds but said I wanted to be with her completely, no matter how long it took. I pass no judgement on what others do in their personal lives, but for me that means no sex workers. I like waking up knowing Mary and the kids get the best of me. I get inner peace living a life where my moral boundaries are now clear.

———

I only really get the treatments that helped me. Nevertheless, everyone needs scaffolding, a framework for their journey out of trauma. My advice is to understand the three stages of treatment and recovery developed in the late 19th century by Pierre Janet, a pioneering French psychotherapist and philosopher. Experts such as American psychiatrist Judith Herman have modified Janet's wording, but his principles remain the same and are straightforward. The stages are an attempt to impose simplicity and order upon a complex process, rather than be taken literally, Herman says.

The stages – and I largely use Herman's wording – are:

1. Establishing safety.
2. Remembrance and mourning, reconstructing the trauma story.
3. Reconnection with ordinary life.

Stage one. Janet focused on stabilisation and symptom reduction; Herman on safety of the survivor, such as surroundings and support networks in the case of rape or domestic violence.

Social support is the most powerful protection against becoming overwhelmed by trauma, says Bessel van der Kolk. 'The critical issue is reciprocity, being truly heard and seen by the people around us. For our physiology to calm down, heal and grow, we need a visceral feeling of safety.'

Adds David Morris: 'One group of VA [Veteran's Administration] researchers, 25 years of research, said the major post traumatic factor is whether a traumatized person received social support. Indeed, receipt of social support, which appears to be the most important factor of all, can protect trauma-exposed individuals from developing PTSD.'

Van der Kolk and Morris are right, but that support must go deep for someone to heal. It must extend into the workplace, be reflected in the availability of psychological services, the creation of a more humane justice system and government departments whose mission is to help people.

Stage one must be established before therapy is attempted.

A combination of factors tipped me into turmoil after my PTSD diagnosis in early 2016: emotional denial about my condition; a psychiatrist in Hobart who didn't get me; social isolation; and indifferent bosses. Then I was a risk to myself. This again illustrates how the real psychological outcome is determined by what happens – or more precisely *doesn't* happen – *after* trauma. Establishing safety began the moment I entered Ward 17. Sure, my anxiety was sky-high, but the intake interviews eased me into accepting I needed hospitalisation. There was no stigma about the word suicide. The building itself was peaceful. I had a private room. Within 24 hours I was sitting across from Maryam. My mind and body felt safe. My treating team could begin to try to stabilise my symptoms.

I didn't realise how useful medication could be in aiding safety and stability until my first Ward 17 admission when Maryam changed my antidepressants, put me on meds for nightmares, and prescribed sleeping tablets and Valium. Medication has worked in the background. Smoothed out my moods, helped me sleep.

It was only after I left Reuters that I had the bandwidth to reflect on Steve Biddulph's advice to listen to my body – a key element to establishing safety. This had been in much of the literature I'd read about trauma, but I didn't get it. My mantra as a journalist was to push through the stress and fatigue, get the job done. Get up the next day and do it again.

I asked Mum in 2020 why she thought I was like that. 'It was in your persona to be driven,' she said. 'And I was old fashioned. I was a slave driver. I can't see the point in living on this earth unless you're there to do something.' Okay Mum!

I knew there were mental health benefits to physical exercise, of walking every day. But I didn't understand what listening to my body really meant. Now I stop and notice tiredness that occasionally extends from my head to my toes; notice anxiety and name it, asking where it's coming from and why, putting my hand on the area. Or stress, which usually manifests in mental wobbles, as if I'm about to tip over and fall to pieces.

PTSD and stress are shocking bedfellows. My threshold for stress is much lower than when I worked overseas in war and disaster zones. I stress easily if I'm rundown, haven't exercised or have been eating too much sugar. Strategies I adopt include taking a break, chopping wood, listening to rock music, sitting in a quiet room, reading a book, having a hot shower, going for a walk, doing something with Mary or watching rugby league matches with Harry. And I always try to keep Mary in the loop. No code words necessary.

All these things, by the way, are what I call mindfulness.

*

Stage two: This means the processing of trauma. I've tried to approach this with curiosity. Constantly questioning my family, my clinicians, friends and former colleagues but especially myself. Reflecting and using deliberate rumination and journaling. You can ask yourself the hardest questions if you write them down. Once I pieced together my role in Namir and Saeed's deaths, I could seek their forgiveness, and forgive myself. The Greek word for purification is *katharsis*, from which we get catharsis, meaning the purification or purging of repressed emotions. That's how I felt walking out of the Anzac Memorial Chapel with Cath after the memorial service for Namir and Saeed – pure release.

Human connections must underpin treatment. You can't do it on your own. Maryam, Cath and Christina helped change the course of my life. They opened their hearts and took the journey with me in Ward 17. Dee and Wendy did it outside. I suspect some practitioners prefer to stay behind walls they call boundaries. It's safer there. Mary came across this great quote when she was counselling refugees: 'I'd rather a therapist with a warm heart and no boundaries than a therapist with a cold heart and firm boundaries.' Of course, no one should take the 'no boundaries' thing literally. But I've seen 25 doctors, psychologists and psychiatrists in the past eight years about my mental state. I know when someone sees me. I feel connection. I can sense a cold heart from a warm one. I know waitlists are horrendous, but if your gut tells you that your therapist doesn't want to take the journey with you, find one who will.

Cath's understanding of the soul lifted a ten-year-old burden off my shoulders. I took part in a panel discussion at the annual conference of Spiritual Care Australia in June 2019 and was struck by the despondency among participants that the medical and psych profession would never see spiritual care workers and chaplains as partners in the treatment of trauma and mental illness. That needs to change.

I sometimes reflect on the group session Cath held in Ward 17 during my third admission in 2018, when she got patients to write down our most important values from a list of more than 100. Cath wasn't telling us how to live our lives. But her simple exercise helped me see I was living the wrong one. It was a big awakening for me. I occasionally pull out those A3 pages with the yellow post-it notes on them and smile.

I've sifted through many experiences and images with my clinicians, with Mary, other times in front of my computer while journaling. I've forced myself to recall the things in my personal life I'm not proud of. When I've gone back to my journals, I've had pleasant discoveries like: *Oh, I used to think like that*, or *Wow, I've made progress there*. This has led to insight. My experiences have become part of my life, my new narrative. They have shaped who I am today, as a husband and a father, and who I want to become tomorrow. This is called integration, a word used by clinicians and written about in trauma books. Namir and Saeed are integrated into my life story, a properly filed memory, albeit a significant one. I don't get stressed when I think or talk about them. They have their own space in my linen cupboard. It doesn't bother me that I could have stopped blaming Namir years ago had I just watched Collateral Murder sooner. That's life. What I'm trying to say here is that dealing with the traumatic experience can be postponed up to a point. But it has to be addressed.

Some things take years to understand when reconstructing your trauma story. One day in 2021, Mary had a revelation about why I couldn't sit with her and Harry in the Singapore hospital after he was born – it reminded me of Bali and the shame of not being able to do my job six weeks earlier. Dee told me later that my body would have rebelled against the hospital smell, the quiet, the surgical gowns, the lighting. It would have wanted to flee that sterile environment.

Because I've worked so hard on my 'recovery', I've sometimes trusted my instincts over the experts. My Ward 17 treating team wanted me to sign a contract to slow down during my first admission. I dismissed the idea as nonsense. I chided senior staff for not having any books on PTSD, trauma or war in the ward library. Why would anyone want to read airport novels, I said, brushing off their concerns that patients might be triggered by the material I was consuming. But just as I did in the field for Reuters, I sometimes pushed myself too hard. The advice to pace myself was good. I should have listened. The more I learnt about trauma, the more I thought I had all the answers. Which is why when Dee said one day she believed the deaths of Namir and Saeed was a PTSD event for me, that moral injury came later, I nearly replied, *No way, it's all moral injury*. It pays to keep an open mind. I had deep respect for Dee, her experience and inter-est in me. She'd been my psychologist for three years by then. We talked it through: traumatic deaths of people I knew and was responsible for (PTSD); watching them about to die when shown the first few minutes of video (vicarious trauma); classic PTSD symptom of avoidance, not wanting to deal with the issue when Julian Assange published Collateral Murder; and the less well-known symptom of self-blame. The moral injury was how I assessed myself as being culpable over their deaths and cowardly for not speaking up publicly. I nodded slowly in agreement. (Maryam later said Dee was correct.)

Driving home that day, I thought: Did that mean ritual, like the memorial service I held for Namir and Saeed in 2017, was a way to treat PTSD? Would I have undertaken such a healing journey if I hadn't been obsessed about moral injury? What this showed was that, whether PTSD or moral injury or a combination of both, I found a way to heal because I made room for guidance.

Stage two has helped me discover self-compassion. After Reuters published my first PTSD special report in late 2016, a group of Iraqi colleagues sent kind messages of support. One wrote: 'Dean saved my life and my family. I feel thanks and gratitude to him. In 2007 I was threatened by al-Qaeda because I worked for Reuters. When Dean heard he told me and my family to leave our house immediately and helped me rent a house for a year and half near the office. We would have been killed if we stayed.'

This message didn't register at the time because I was so focused on reckoning with myself over Namir and Saeed. I didn't refer to this man's circumstances in the note I wrote for Maryam in Ward 17 a few months earlier on the good things I'd done for staff because I had no memory of it. Yet it was one of the most important I'd done in my life.

I show myself compassion all the time now because I've done the work to warrant it. People are quick to say to others: it wasn't your fault; it's not your responsibility. But what if it was, totally or partly? What if being told to be kind to yourself is the last thing someone wants to hear? Next time you hear someone talk like this, think before you speak. Maybe that person wants validation, support, or even better for someone to say: 'Tell me your story. I'm ready to listen.'

Stage three. Reconnection with ordinary life. My old friend Andrew Marshall laid the foundation before my first Ward 17 admission when he told me I wasn't alone. A few months later I was inundated with messages of support after Reuters published my special report. And so, I began rebuilding my sense of self, writing my new narrative. I reconnected with old friends, made new ones.

The most important reconnection, of course, was with Mary and my kids.

Western societies make it hard for trauma survivors to reconnect with ordinary life because we isolate and shame them. We don't encourage them to share their story. Or when they do in the case of sexual assault, right-wing commentators and politicians try to tear them down. We miss out on their wisdom. It initially surprised me how much the patients in Ward 17 wanted to talk to me about their experiences. Then I realised it was because no one listens. We need to let trauma survivors speak so we can communalise their pain. War, natural disasters and sexual violence are the same the world over. What is different is how communities respond. When survivors are shunned and stigmatised, their journeys back are so much harder.

Some people express surprise when I tell them that every veteran and first responder I know would do their job again. They'd put on the uniform in a heartbeat, get behind the wheel of an ambulance, jump into a fire truck or strap a service revolver to their waist. I'd grab my notepad and catch a plane to the breaking news. It's good to remind ourselves of this because our missions had meaning. Viktor Frankl was right. People need to strive for a worthwhile goal. I've found meaning in the three ways he wrote about: creating a work (writing); loving another person (Mary and my kids); and turning what I went through into a life filled with purpose.

My journey shows that recovery is not a straight line and that these three stages can occur out of sequence. I guarantee there will be setbacks. Those have been learning opportunities for me, a chance to reset.

Dee Cooper likens recovery to the centuries-old Japanese art of Kintsugi, or Kintsukuroi, the use of lacquer mixed with powdered metals to repair broken or chipped pottery. Picture a large bowl held together with veins of gold-coloured lacquer. The bowl is intact, fully usable, but scarred. It's a wonderful way to think about trauma because we're all fractured in some way. We shouldn't be ashamed of the cracks because they represent survival. The scarring makes us unique.

Author's note

My extensive journals, as well as emails and other documents form the bedrock of the sourcing in my memoir. When I use someone's full name, that means they've agreed to be identified and have checked the material to make sure it's accurate. Some people only wanted their first name used, or a pseudonym. Those people also signed off on what I wrote.

Acknowledgements

My partner Mary Binks has been the biggest supporter of this book from the start. She encouraged me to write it even before I felt I had a story to share. No one wants to read another book by a former foreign correspondent, I'd say. But Mary also knew this book would test us because she thought more deeply about our relationship than I did at the time.

Thank you, Mary, for everything.

Patrick, Belle and Harry deserve medals for putting up with me. I can't begin to imagine how difficult it's been for them. I dreaded telling them about my infidelity to Mary. They've forgiven me too. They've seen me get better, forge a new life, and that doesn't always happen for children whose parents have PTSD. As Harry said to me in early 2023, one dad went into Ward 17, another one came out. That spoke to me of the transformation I've undergone.

I first met Jeremy Wagstaff in 1993 in Jakarta where he was working for Reuters. I joined later that year. Our paths crossed at various points in Asia. Jeremy checked on me virtually every day in 2016. Mary sought his advice when I wouldn't listen to her. When she needed to talk about how awful things were for our family. Or when she needed to laugh. (It was the same with Jeremy's wife Sari Sudarsono and our other friend from Indonesia, Tessa Piper.)

Reuters Asia made Jeremy redundant at the end of 2017, said his job was no longer needed. I wonder if there was an element of payback from Reuters Asia in sacking Jeremy because he kept pushing them to help me. I sent the angriest email I've ever written to top management in New York when he was fired. It made no difference and Reuters never formally acknowledged the lengths he went to in keeping me alive.

Author Tom Ricks has been a big supporter of my writing on trauma since he read my first PTSD special report in late 2016 and has generously introduced me to various people in the United States.

Steve Biddulph helped me understand that my PTSD would have long-lasting consequences for Mary, Patrick, Belle and Harry. He always responded thoughtfully to my emails, offered his expertise. When Patrick was in grade 11, having just turned seventeen, and announced he wanted to quit school to focus on his art, Steve calmed me down.

Some years ago, I asked Steve if he might endorse a children's book written by a colleague's wife. I mentioned I was making progress on mine but was frustrated trying to find an agent. The global literary agency I was speaking to didn't seem interested, didn't understand how widespread trauma was, nor get what a curious journalist with lived experience could do with the subject, I said. A high-profile agent in New York whom Tom Ricks had introduced me to said he didn't think the book would work for a general interest publisher. The ABC's Leigh Sales had told me publishers were wary of what she called dark subjects, but keep trying to find an agent, she advised. All this made me worried and a little depressed, I said to Steve in an email, asking for his thoughts. Steve said he'd decline reading the children's book because he gets so many requests. 'But YOUR book is a different story,' he wrote.

So began Steve's mentoring of me on this project, which ranged from telling me not to call workers' comp insurers scumbags to challenging me over a paragraph in which I said I had a great childhood. I was never abused in any way, never bullied at school, I was popular, good at sport, that sort of thing, I'd written. 'Dean – there is adversity in all childhoods,' Steve said. 'There is much emotional repression in what we call normal Western childhoods. Most children come to adulthood with considerable impairment, which is why trauma is handled so badly.' Steve also gave me great writing advice. Imagine the page is a piece of wood, and you're holding an old-fashioned planer. Plane that wood until it's perfectly smooth, he said. In other words, keep writing, re-writing and editing.

Professor Alexander (Sandy) McFarlane has contributed enormously to the global understanding of trauma in military and civilian contexts. Like Steve, I'm proud to call Sandy a friend. Sandy and I clicked the first time we met in early 2017 in Melbourne, after I'd been to Ward 17 with the documentary filmmakers and felt so sick I wasn't sure I could interview him. I've spoken to Sandy countless times about PTSD, veterans and first responders. Sandy ran the Centre for Traumatic Stress Studies (CTSS) at Adelaide University until it was forced to close in late 2019. The CTSS had been one of the best trauma research facilities in the world. But it had to shut when the Australian Defence Force and the Department of Veterans' Affairs, its two biggest financial backers for a decade, halted funding. Sandy had worked closely with the ADF and DVA for three decades. He never got a straight answer on why the financial taps were turned off, but I suspect it was partly because the government of then Prime Minister Scott Morrison didn't like independent experts at CTSS showing how badly veterans were suffering from PTSD and other mental illnesses.

I'm extremely grateful to people around the world who read the entire manuscript or parts, either to fact-check sections if they were identified or were asked for their view:

Ward 17 staff and patients: Sean Callaghan, Jo Donovan, Lieutenant-Colonel (retired) Karel Dubsky, Stewart Hulls, Adrian Jallands, Brett Lewindon, Dr Maryam, Christina Sim, Soldier D, Soldier J, Matt Ross, Cath Taylor, Ray Watson.

Current and former Reuters staff: Carlos Barria, Luke Baker, Beawiharta, Edmund Blair, Erik de Castro, Andy Cawthorne, Gina Chua, Jo Collins, Ross Colvin, Steve Crisp, Guy Desmond, Adam Entous, Alix Freedman, Minami Funakoshi, Matthew Green, Girish Gupta, Chris Helgren, Paul Holmes, Aseel Kami, Mariam Karouny, Francis Kerry, Ciara Lee, Michael Lawrence, Alastair Macdonald, Andrew Marshall, Rodney Pinder, Anne-Marie Roantree, David Schlesinger, Tomi Soejipto, Paul Tait, Mehreen Zahra-Malik and Mike Williams. Also, Baghdad security advisors Sam Jamison and Bill Jervis. I'm not sure I would have lasted if it wasn't for their support, and the tea and biscuits they offered when I sought sanctuary in their tidy office on the second floor of our newsroom in the Iraqi capital.

Other journalists: Chris Booth, Paul Daley, Caroline Hawley, Chris Hedges, Allison Jackson, David Leser, Lisa Millar, Hugh Riminton, Manuela Saragosa and Journalist YZ, not to be confused with Journalists AZ and DZ. YZ, I will tell more of your story another time.

Others who have read all or parts of the book: Sharyn Anderson, Michael 'Doc' Bailey, John Bale, Helen Barrow, Chris Binks, Michael Bradley, Dee Cooper, Dr Mark Cross, Fiora, Wendy Gall, Professor Sam Harvey, Mick Halloran, Vanessa Heuser, Dr Sadhbh Joyce, Bree Knoester, Tara Lal, Jacqui Lambie, Professor Brett Litz, Hanabeth Luke, Gabriel Mac, Geoff McDonald, Dr Polly McGee, Amy McKeown, Cait McMahon, Simon Philips, Clothilde Redfern, Terry Reid, Professor Nancy Sherman, Edward Tick, Nick Todhunter, Sophie Todhunter, Kate Tunstall, Jamie Watson, Peter Whish-Wilson, Kim Williams, Simone Whetton, Holly Yates and my parents Pam Sainsbury and John Yates.

A general shout-out to other Ward 17 patients: Rob Atkins, Bob Breakspear, Annika Field, Abbie-lee Hamilton, Greg Fordham, Sue Cooper, Rob Jordan, Ben McAllister, Ian Blake, Sam Scheske and staff Tracey Kenny, Anne Poole and Maya Seoud.

David Fox, an old Reuters colleague and former inmate of Bali's Kerobokan jail, shared some of my journey. I couldn't find room in this book for our story David, but I will at some point.

My old Sydney University mates and walking buddies have been an immense support. Thank you Guy Boland, Matt Burgess, Saul Duffy, Paul Goldman, Dale Greer, Mick Halloran, Patrick McCormack, Paul Scott, Tim Stanley, Nick Todhunter, Phil Towzell and Damien Tynan.

I was proud to work for Reuters for 26 years, whether in the field, in a newsroom calling a government official or working on a desk editing a story. I loved the company's reputation for accuracy. I loved the way we threw everything at the big stories. Working in a team was everything for me: I'll always remember the drivers in Baghdad who – like Saeed Chmagh – risked their lives every day; the Vietnamese staff who wrote coffee reports one day and covered devastating floods the next; Indonesian photographers and TV staff who captured that amazing country in all its mystery, colour and agony; the graphics journalists in Singapore who showed me there was yet another way to tell a story. And a special mention to Reuters colleagues everywhere who cover anything that moves a financial market. I worked hard to stay away from those sorts of stories because I didn't have the nerve. Baghdad, yes. Financial markets, no.

My publisher Cate Blake made clear from the get-go she wanted me at Pan Macmillan and nowhere else. I didn't have to explain moral injury to her, she got it. Cate also asked some big questions that forced me to reflect on things that, while making me uncomfortable, had to be done. Editor Rebecca Lay combined organisational and production calm with sound advice at a time when looming deadlines had my heart racing. Copyeditor Susin Chow did a masterful job helping Dean the journalist (hopefully) complete the transition to Dean the author.

Unlike most copyeditors I've worked with, too, Susin was polite about virtually every change she wanted to make. Publicist Allie Schotte brought youth, energy and ideas to the campaign, getting me opportunities across the board. Pan's Marketing Executive Rufus Cuthbert introduced me to a book trailer, something I didn't know existed. Thank you also to my agent Gaby Naher at Left Bank Literary, for her tireless work in finding me the right publisher. And Paul Daley at *The Guardian* for introducing me to Gaby.

On a balmy Saturday evening in early March 2023, I sat on the stage of the Great Hall at Sydney University; the twentieth anniversary of the US-led invasion of Iraq was two weeks away. Nearly twenty people were giving testimony live and via video under the banner of the Belmarsh Tribunal as to why Julian Assange should be released and reunited with his family. It would be the *first* time I'd have the opportunity to present publicly the facts of Chapter 20: Rules of engagement. The Great Hall was full, and the event was being streamed live. I'm an experienced public speaker but I was nervous. Tightness gripped my chest. I spilt water on myself as I got up to speak and then over my notes on the lectern. All day I'd thought to myself: what if my speech really upsets people. And by people, I meant the United States. *That* is the chilling effect of the persecution and prosecution of Julian Assange. Which is why I salute his courage and that of Chelsea Manning in risking everything by exposing US lies about the war in Iraq and what really happened to Namir Noor-Eldeen and Saeed Chmagh.

Finally, I pay my deepest respects to the families of Namir, Saeed and Lu'oy al-Joubouri. May those three men rest in peace.